Reverse Prediabetes, Diabetes, Fatty Liver and Lose Weight

How to Achieve Your Goal and Maintain it Affordably

By

Shunzhong Shawn Bao, MD

Editor: Barbara Winter

Ace Health Publisher

Publisher's Note: The information contained herein is not intended to replace the services of a trained health professional or to be a substitute for individual medical advice. You should consult with your health care professional in regard to any matter relating to your health, and in particular, any matter that may require diagnosis or medical attention. If you are being treated for diabetes, any changes in your existing medications are not advised without first consulting a medical professional. Additionally, any changes in your diet and exercise practices should follow the guidelines of a medical professional who has personally examined you and reviewed your records.

Reverse Prediabetes, Diabetes, Fatty Liver and Lose Weight
How to Achieve Your Goal and Maintain it Affordably

Shunzhong Shawn Bao, M.D.
Barbara Winter, Editor

Published by: Ace Health Publisher

Preface

We all know obesity is a major problem for the modern world, and we have hundreds of books being written trying to help people lose weight. There are countless diets and programs. People are jumping from one diet to another. Talking about the long-term effect, it is abysmal. This is why so many people are seeking medications, some even illegally and also as the last resort-surgery.

Most diets use one group of macronutrients to replace another macronutrient group. Fat was replaced by carbs; and now carbs are being replaced by fats and/or proteins.

I know you will want to follow the recommendations I have in this book. The idea I talk about is not just about losing weight but living better and improving your health.

I know you can do it. The recommendations I give in this book are simple, affordable and working. I have many patients who were able to follow my simple recommendations and thus able to lose 10 lbs, 20 lbs, 50 lbs and even 100 lbs. I have patients who reversed their prediabetes, fatty liver disease and even diabetes. I did a survey among my patients who had 20% of body weight loss and kept it off for two years. Overwhelmingly my patients said my recommendations are really easy to follow and work. People are also improving their skills of managing their stress while improving their emotional intelligence.

Eating is a basic need for surviving and is primarily regulated by the hypothalamus which is unaware to us. However, our prefrontal lobe is more powerful and can consciously adjust and change the course of hypothalamus commands. In this book, I promote balanced and diverse whole foods. You are not deprived of a whole group of food, nor required to buy expensive packaged food. You will eat better!

The big substage force for prefrontal lobe power is stress. This book brings you the good way to improve your skill of dealing with stress. I discuss all major stress sources, namely stress from the workplace (job, boss, colleagues), stress from family (spouse, parents, children) and stress from financial concerns.

This book is straightforward and uses language with which you are familiar. The recommendations are also very practical and easy to follow. The most important thing is that they work. I have tried them on hundreds of patients. This book is good for anyone who wants to live better and be healthier without obesity, prediabetes, diabetes, or fatty liver disease.

Dedication

This book is dedicated to my patients. These are their intelligent questions for which I am grateful. They motivate me to think, continue learning and improve my patient care every day. These days, doctors struggle to address all the questions patients may have. I hope my patients will get some answers here.

I want to thank my nurses, Betty Westbury and Michelle Nevener, who are providing excellent care to my patients and were the first readers of this book. With their critiques, they have made significant contributions.

This book is also dedicated to my good friend, my editor, Barbara Winter, for her unending kindness and generosity. With her patience and critical editing, she has made this book readable.

Finally, this book is dedicated to my wife who deserves deep, enduring gratitude, and also to my two children who are both in medical school. They are "first round editors". They helped me despite their heavy medical school work. They inspire me to learn and strive for excellence in patient care.

Contents

Chapter 1. Diagnosis of Obesity, Fatty Liver Prediabetes and Diabetes

Questions about an obesity diagnosis

How do I know if I am overweight or obese?

Now obesity is a disease, and we can make the diagnosis of obesity. Unfortunately, most insurance companies still do not pay for obesity management. Most clinicians make the diagnosis of obesity using BMI (body mass index) as criteria since it is easy and simple. Busy clinicians do not need extra work. It is also very simple for patients to understand, assess, and monitor themselves.

What are the BMI criteria to make the diagnosis of obesity?

The following is the BMI criteria for the general population. For Asians, the criteria are slightly different. BMI is short for body mass index which can be calculated using the formula: body mass in kilogram divided by the square of the body height in meters. You can just google an online calculator to figure out your BMI. If you are under care of a doctor, you can just ask your doctor. It is automatically generated in your chart.

Overweight: 25-29.9
Class I : 30-34.9
Class II: 35-39.9
Class III: 40 or greater
Class III sometimes is also referred to as morbid obesity. Again, Asians have lower criteria. I consider >37.5 as morbid obesity for Asians.

What should we take into consideration when we apply the BMI criteria?

We should practice caution in applying the BMI criteria to you if you:

- Have significant fluid retention
- Are an athlete with significant muscle mass
- Have a large tumor. I saw a lady for something else and found she had an extended abdomen. I ordered an ultrasound. She was found to have a 20 lb ovarian tumor.
- Are Asians since there is slightly different criteria.

What else can you do to assess my “fatness”?

We also have a waist circumference criterion, bioelectric impedance, air/water displacement plethysmography, or dual-energy x-ray absorptiometry, ultrasound, CT or MRI. In clinic, the circumference is easy to do. The rest costs more money and usually it is not necessary.

What is the waist circumference (WC) criteria?

Many different organizations set up many different criteria. The following is what I go by.

Country or ethnic group	Central obesity as defined by WC	
	Men - inches (cm)	**Women - inches (cm)**
European, Sub-Saharan African, Eastern Mediterranean and Middle Eastern (Arab)	40 (102) or greater	35 (88) or greater
South Asian, Chinese, Japanese, South and Central American	36 (90) or greater	32 (80) or greater

Should I measure my own waist circumference?

You should. The more attention you pay to your weight, the better you will be. I encourage my patients to monitor themselves.

How is waist circumference measured?

1. Remove clothing from the waist line.
2. Stand with feet and shoulders in a line.
3. Locate the top of the hip bone at the side. Use the area between the thumb and index finger to feel for the hip bone at the side of the waist.
4. Align the bottom edge of the measuring tape with the top of the hip bone. Wrap the tape measure all the way around the waist. Ensure that the tape measure is parallel to the floor and not twisted.
5. Take two normal breaths and on the exhale of the second breath tighten the tape measure so it is snug but not digging into the skin.
6. Take the measure of the waist to the nearest 0.5 cm (1/4 inch).
7. Repeat two or three times and calculate the average.

Questions about obesity complications

What is prediabetes?

Blood sugar is not normal, but it does not reach the diagnosis of diabetes yet. Specifically,

- fasting sugar is between 100-125 mg /dl
- oral glucose testing, two-hour sugar between 140-199
- HbA1c is between 5.7%-6.4%.

Can prediabetes have the same complications as diabetes?

Yes. People with prediabetes can develop complications. The diagnosis of diabetes is arbitrary. The changes in our body are a continuous process and form a spectrum.

Should I test for prediabetes?

You should. 30% of adult Americans have prediabetes and 90% of them do not know about it. When you know it, you can do something about it. You will be better. Next time, when you see your doctor, please ask about it.

What is diabetes?

The diagnostic criteria are when any items exceed the cut-off for prediabetes (see above question for prediabetes).

As I stated in my first diabetes book (Google my name or search my name on Amazon.com), diabetes is defined as high sugar in the blood. High sugar in the blood is just a sign. Strictly, diabetes should not be a standalone diagnosis. There are many reasons. In the current medical community, we have type 1 and type 2 diabetes. In reality, we have a dozen reasons which can cause sugar to increase in the blood. In that sense, we have a dozen different types of diabetes. So, when we give people a diagnosis of diabetes, we should also give the possible cause. Here is an example. You have fever and cough and go to the ER. You are admitted to the hospital. The doctor initially gives you the diagnosis of pneumonia, but the doctor should do his or her best to find what bacteria causes your pneumonia.

For diabetes, you deserve to know the cause so the cause can be treated. Now we lump everyone into two categories, type 1 and type 2 diabetes. You deserve to you more details.

However, for the majority of type 2 diabetes, the cause is over eating in relative to your activity. It is a lifestyle disease. Just like treating pneumonia, we give you oxygen if your oxygenation is compromised; we give you hydration if you are dehydrated; we give you antipyretic like Tylenol if you have high fever. But the most important treatment we give you are the antibiotics to kill the bacteria, and the more specific the better.

If your cause for your diabetes (high blood sugar) is because of over eating supply in blood. You need to change your lifestyle or get rid of some sugar and fat from your body. If not, it is like treating your pneumonia with Tylenol or oxygen. Your pneumonia eventually will get worse and you might die. It is the same thing with your diabetes. It will get worse and worse if we do not treat the cause.

What is the risk for diabetes and prediabetes?

Diabetes is complicated. There are many causes of diabetes. However, for type 2 diabetes, obesity goes hand in hand with it. 90% of type 2 diabetics are overweight or obese. The rest could be misdiagnosed as type 2. Recently, my son, under the guidance of a Washington University professor, reported that type I diabetes is more prevalent in adults than in children. In other words, some type 1 diabetes in adults is misdiagnosed as type 2.

Does lifestyle modification and metformin reduce my risk of developing diabetes?

The Diabetes Prevention Program reported that metformin alone can reduce diabetes risk by 31%, and the combination of intensive lifestyle changes and metformin can reduce the risk by 58%.

What can I do if I am diagnosed with prediabetes/diabetes?

- Read this book carefully to see what you can do in terms of changing your lifestyle.
- Ask your doctor to see if you have certain conditions which cause diabetes. These conditions are, but are not limited to fatty liver, hypothyroidism, Cushing's disease, Acromegaly…
- Ask your doctor to see if you are taking medications which promote weight gain and thus are causing diabetes. The most notorious medications are steroids.
- I make sure you do not have type 1 diabetes.

What is hypertriglyceridemia?

We all know what cholesterol is. Triglycerides are simply the most common fat we see. It is very common and associated with obesity and diabetes. Over nutrition can cause high triglycerides in the blood.

- Normal – <150 mg/dL
- Mild hypertriglyceridemia – 150 to 499 mg/dL
- Moderate hypertriglyceridemia – 500 to 886 mg/dL
- Very high or severe hypertriglyceridemia – >886 mg/dL

What is the risk for moderate hypertriglyceridemia?

The major concern for most patients who have triglycerides over 500 is acute pancreatitis. The cardiovascular risks are complicated by other factors and have not been agreed in detail by the medical community.

What is the typical dyslipidemia in obesity?

As we know, dyslipidemia is the single most modifiable risk factor for cardiovascular disease. The typical dyslipidemia of obesity consists of increased triglycerides (TG) and free fatty acids (FFA), decreased HDL-C (referred to as good cholesterol) with HDL dysfunction and normal or slightly increased LDL-C (referred to as bad cholesterol) with increased small dense LDL (referred to as really bad cholesterol). The concentration of plasma apolipoprotein (apo) B (the carrier of bad cholesterol) is also often increased, partly due to the hepatic overproduction of apoB containing lipoproteins.

What is the risk for hypertension in obesity?

It was estimated that excess body weight (including overweight and obesity) accounted for approximately 26 percent of cases of hypertension in men and 28 percent in women.

What is the risk for coronary heart disease?

Overweight and obesity are responsible for approximately 23 percent of the cases of coronary heart disease in men and 15 percent in women. This does not account for heart failure.

What is the risk for nonalcoholic fatty liver disease?

In the US general population, two-thirds are overweight or obese. 50% of these people have nonalcoholic fatty liver disease. Now nonalcoholic fatty liver disease is the number one cause of cirrhosis.

What is the risk for biliary tract stones (gallstones)?

It is well known that obesity increases the risk for gallstones. Most people believe that obesity increases the synthesis and secretion of cholesterol. I think obesity also causes the dysfunction of the gallbladder. Some research revealed that obesity triples the risk for gallstones. A report about morbid obesity patients reveals that more than 60% have gallstones.

Most obese patients have tried to lose weight and some patients go to extremes like starving or semi-starving to cause rapid weight loss. This way of weight loss also increases the stone formation.

Does obesity cause acid reflux?

Obesity is associated with acid reflux and it is believed to be one of the common causes. The prevalence of acid reflux is increased along the rate of obesity. Obesity is also associated with Barret's esophagus and esophageal cancer.

What is the risk for polycystic ovarian syndrome?

Polycystic ovarian syndrome might cause weight gain and obesity which makes polycystic ovarian syndrome much worse. This is likely a vicious cycle. The exact risk is not very clear. Generally, 10% of women have polycystic ovarian syndrome.

Polycystic ovarian syndrome (PCOS), a heterogeneous, complex genetic trait of unclear etiology, is an important cause of ovulatory and menstrual irregularity (irregular periods, missing periods), subfertility and infertility, clinically evident hyperandrogenism (excessive hair growth, hair loss, excessive acne), and metabolic dysfunction (hypertension, obesity, hyperlipidemia, pre-diabetes, diabetes) in women.

What is the risk for female infertility and pregnancy complications?

Infertility is the lack of pregnancy despite regular unprotected sexual intercourse after a year or therapeutic donor insemination in women less than 35 years of age, and after six months in women 35 years and older.

In several studies, it is found that the risk of infertility is threefold higher in obese women than in non-obese women. It has been shown that the probability of pregnancy is reduced by 5% per unit of BMI exceeding 29 kg/m2.

As we know, obesity causes female hormone imbalance which leads to anovulation (is when the ovaries do not release an oocyte during a menstrual cycle).

Because of reduced pregnancy rates, increased miscarriage rates, and increased pregnancy complications (like preeclampsia, eclampsia), live birth rates decrease in obese women in both natural and assisted conceptions.

What is the prevalence of female obesity at fertile age?

In the United States, National Center for Health Statistics data for 2011 to 2014 indicated that 34 percent of women aged 20 to 39 years were obese; the prevalence was highest in non-Hispanic black women (57 percent). Among US women with live births in 2015, another database indicated that 26 percent were obese pre-pregnancy and another 26 percent were overweight.

What is the risk for obese women with pregnancy?

- The pregnancy loss is increased by more than 30%.
- The rate of diabetes is significantly increased.
- For every 1 kg/m_2 increase in BMI over 25, the rate for gestational diabetes increases by 0.92 percent.
- Morbidity and mortality are both increased significantly.

What is the risk for male hypogonadism?

Many studies show that obesity increases the risk for male hypogonadism. From the European Male Aging Study (EMAS), obesity was associated with an 8.7-fold and overweight with a 3.3-fold increased relative risk (RR) of secondary hypogonadism. Both total testosterone and free testosterone levels were lower in obese compared to lean men, with lesser but still significant reduction in overweight men.

There is a report on US community-dwelling, obese US American men showing 40% had low testosterone levels. If with diabetes also, the rate of low testosterone increased to 57%.

What is the potential mechanism responsible for low testosterone in obese men?

Testosterone is being converted to estrogen at fat cells. The more fat mass you have, the more testosterone is converted to estrogen. The increased estrogen then suppresses your pituitary gland to produce gonadotropins (hormones that stimulate the testicles to produce testosterone). Obesity might also directly affect the testicle function.

Low testosterone causes fatigue, causes fat to grow and then patients gain more weight. Obesity causes obstructive sleep apnea and then leads to lower testosterone. This can be a vicious cycle.

Is there any good news about obesity-induced male hypogonadism?

The good news is that: Obesity-caused male hypogonadism is not permanent. If obesity is reversed, male testosterone is back to normal.

What is the risk for obstructive sleep apnea?

Obstructive sleep apnea is causing major problems in modern society. This is one of the most common causes of fatigue, daytime sleepiness, poor memory, depression, moodiness, low sex drive, and performance. Obstructive sleep apnea also causes weight gain like a self-propelled vicious cycle.

In a community-based cohort of middle-aged subjects, it showed that a single standard deviation increase in BMI was associated with a fourfold increased risk for prevalent sleep apnea. We have demonstrated a sleep apnea prevalence of approximately 40% in moderately overweight men from the community who are otherwise healthy. In severe obesity (BMI > 40 kg/m2), the prevalence of sleep apnea was estimated to vary between 40 and 90%, and the severity of sleep apnea was generally greater than that found in leaner clinical populations. In addition, there is a link between sleep apnea and obesity: a 10% change in body weight was associated with a parallel change of approximately 30% in the apnea–hypopnea index (AHI).

Therefore, anybody with obesity needs screening for obstructive sleep apnea.

What is the risk for other respiratory system conditions?

Obesity can cause other respiratory system issues like increased risk for asthma, deep vein thrombosis (can travel to the lung and cause pulmonary embolism), reduced lung volume and restrictive dysfunction, or reduced lung and chest compliance.

Questions about fatty liver disease

What is nonalchoholic fatty liver disease (NAFLD)?

Basically, there is too much fat accumulated in the liver cells and not caused by too much alcohol. The accumulated fat can cause the liver to not function properly and can also cause inflammation (hepatitis). The inflammation can cause cell death and leads to scar formation which is cirrhosis.

Therefore, if we use a different pathology to classify nonalchoholic fatty liver disease, we can classify it into fatty liver (no inflammation), nonalcoholic steatohepatitis (NASH), and cirrhosis. Usually if you have inflammation, you have different degrees of cirrhosis.

How common is the NAFLD?

There is a big database called NHANES. They made the diagnosis based on increased liver enzymes but non-alcohol intake. The prevalence rate was increased progressively. We know this is underestimated. There are many people who have fatty liver, but the liver enzymes are still normal

In a study of 400 US military personnel (they are relatively healthier than the general population) and their families (mean age 55 years), the prevalence of NAFLD by ultrasound was 46 percent.

The data is really alarming.

This is not only happening in America. This trend is happening around the world. Some third world countries are catching up fast.

Some Asian countries are already reported to have NAFLD as high as 35%.

What are the dangers for NAFLD?

NAFLD has been suggested to causes:

- diabetes.
- dyslipidemia.
- abnormal liver enzymes leading to much more testing.
- increased blood pressure.
- cardiovascular disease.

- liver cirrhosis.
- liver cancer.
- susceptibility to hepatitis virus infection.
- reduced life expectancy by 10-15 years.

What is the cause of NAFLD?

Although the exact cause and pathogenesis are still not very clear, the very close correlation of obesity and type 2 diabetes make us think they might have the same cause- which is the nutrition overload and sedentarism.

Increased sugar increase liver to produce more fat. Increased inflammation in the fat cells increase liver to store fat more. Unhealthy diet causes gut dysbiosis (the gut flora depleted or not balanced), a leaky gut, microorganism derived products causing liver inflammation, fat storage and fibrosis.

What are the most common symptoms of NAFLD?

The most common symptoms are no symptoms. Some patients might have upper right abdominal discomfort and fatigue.

How do we make the diagnosis of NAFLD?

The diagnosis of NAFLD is one of exclusion and assumption for some cases. If needed, we confirm the diagnosis by biopsy.

First, we confirm that you have fatty liver disease by imaging (most common- ultrasound, MRI) and biopsy.
Biopsy is the ultimate diagnostic tool.

Second, exclude moderate to excessive alcohol use.

Third, exclude other common or uncommon causes if needed for liver disease, like virus hepatitis, hemochromatosis (too much iron). Wilson disease (too much copper), alpha-1 antitrypsin deficiency, etc.

Fourth, exclude some medications and other conditions which might cause abnormal liver enzymes like severe hypothyroidism, or celiac disease.

Liver biopsy is scary. Do I really need it?

Again, the liver biopsy is the gold standard for determining fibrosis/the severity of the disease.

There are many indices which were developed to help doctors to assess the need for biopsy, e.g. FIB-4 index using AST, platelet count, ALT and age; NAFLD fibrosis score (NFS) using age, BMI (body mass index), presence of prediabetes/diabetes, albumin, platelet count, AST and ALT level; or just AST to platelet ratio index score. There is also a patented mathematical formula that takes into account age, sex and levels of gamma-glutamyl transferase, total bilirubin, haptoglobin, apolipoprotein-A, and alpha-2 macroglobulin.

If possible, doctors also use non-invasive imaging to assess your liver fibrosis. Ultrasound is used often. Doctors assess your liver "transient elastography" using a special transducer. They can also assess acoustic radiation force imaging to assess your liver stiffness. MRI elastography is being used more and more often because it is clearer and more accurate.
What I do is to calculate the NAFLD fibrosis score (NFS). If the score is greater than -1.455, then I refer the patient to a liver specialist. If you do the FIB-4 score, the cutoff is 1.3.

What can I do if I am diagnosed with NAFLD?

We do not have a magic medication yet.

We know if you can correct the nutrition overload, the early stage of NAFLD can be reversed. This is really good news. Start today and now. Follow this book's recommendations: start to eat healthier, exercise and manage your stress better.

What are the cancers which are strongly associated with overweight and obesity?

More cancers are being added to the following list:

- Endometrial (uterine)
- Kidney
- Gastric (stomach)
- Colon
- Rectum
- Biliary tract

- Pancreas
- Breast (in women who had never taken hormones)
- Esophageal adenocarcinoma
- Ovarian
- Multiple myeloma
- Hepatocellular carcinoma
- Meningioma
- Prostate
- And more

Obesity and overweight also increase the likelihood of dying from cancer. The American Cancer Society warned that obesity would be the number one preventable cause for cancer in the near future. Now smoking is still the number one preventable cause.

Do we know the mechanism for which obesity causes cancer?

Scientists are still working day and night in elucidating the exact link. We already know some of them. The obesity causes the insulin and insulin-like factors to increase. They are the growth factors which promote cancer growth. Obesity also causes sick fat cells which secrete inflammatory factors and also cause cancer to occur and grow.

Why does obesity cause low extremity swelling?

People with obesity have a much higher rate of low extremity swelling for the following reason. Obesity has been indicated to cause

- increased venous system pressure
- venous system insufficiency
- lymphedema
- heart failure
- deep vein thrombosis (DVT)

Why does obesity cause DVT?

The risk for DVT is more than doubled in obese patients. Obesity increases the risk for DVT and potential other risk factors such as Leiden V mutation, immobility, smoking, taking an oral contraceptive, having antiphospholipid antibodies, etc. to cause DVT.

Obesity and arthritis, which is “the egg”, which is “the chicken”?

Most people would agree with me, obesity is the chicken producing the arthritis in this relationship. The fat mass causes joint cartilage damage leading to arthritis. Arthritis is such a debilitating condition which causes a lot of pain, and immobility. This certainly can cause more weight gain.

Many patients have knee or hip replacements in their life time. Many patients end up with substance abuse due to the pain.

Do obese patients have a higher risk for gout?

Gout is caused by the precipitation of uric acid (urate) in the soft tissues or joints which causes inflammation and results in severe pain. The risk of developing gouty arthritis increases with body weight and with the amount of weight gain during adulthood.

Is obesity a risk factor for urinary incontinence?

Yes, the obesity increases the incontinence rate significantly in women.

Why do obese people have a higher rate of renal failure?

Obesity increases other conditions which cause renal (kidney) failure such as hypertension and diabetes. There are also some hormonal changes which lead to renal failure.

Do obese people have a higher rate of kidney stones?

Both calcium-based stones and urate-based stones are increased.

Why does obesity cause depression?

Obesity is tough. It is why I emphasize obesity prevention. I monitor every single patient’s weight even if they have perfect weight. I always let them know we all need to know our weight and be vigilant. It is very easy for us to gain weight but very difficult to lose weight.

These are the possible reasons causing depression:

- Obesity causes social stigma. Obesity is a disease, but it is perceived as laziness and lack of self-control.
- Obesity reduces people's self-confidence which might lead to social isolation.
- People are working and starving to lose weight but fail. Most people have very frustrating weight loss experiences.
- Obesity can cause complications. Those complications/sickness can also pull people down.
- Obesity causes more sick days which might reduce pay which cause additional difficulties.
- Obesity also brings hormonal changes which might be implicated in depression.

Dose obesity cause headaches?

Obesity is known to be associated with migraine and other headaches.

Why does obesity have higher risk for dementia?

Obesity has a higher rate for dementia for the following reasons:

- Obesity has more negative emotions like depression, stress, anxiety.
- Obesity can lead to social isolation.
- Obesity can have complications like hypertension, atrial fibrillation, or diabetes which lead to stroke and then to dementia.
- Obesity can cause chronic headaches which are associated with dementia.
- Obesity has reduced physical activity which is associated with dementia.
- Obese patients are taking more medications. Polypharmacy is associated with dementia.

Why are obese patients more susceptible to infection?

Obese patients are more susceptible to all sorts of infections including influenzas. The infections are more severe and more likely to require hospitalization and possibly end in death.

The exact reason is not very clear. There is no concrete evidence to show that the immune system is weak in obese patients. Here are a few reasons I can think of:

- Obesity weakens the point of entry for bacteria and viruses.
- Obesity can harbor some bacteria in the skin folds.
- Obesity can be complicated by renal failure, liver disease and diabetes which can weaken the immunity.
- Obesity can lead to more health care facility visits which expose the person to more bacteria and viruses.
- As we discussed above, obesity cause stress/depression which might weaken the immune system.
- Obesity has a higher level of inflammation which also might weaken your immunity.

What are the skin changes in obesity?

Obesity can also cause skin changes:

- Skin infection. All sorts skin infections are increased and much more severe. Infection in the axillar and groin area can be very severe.
- Obesity and diabetes are also associated with Fourier gangrene (private parts deep infection-very severe condition.)
- Stretch marks (striae) are common and reflect the tension on the skin from expanding subcutaneous deposits of fat.
- Acanthosis nigricans, with deepening pigmentation around the neck, axilla, knuckles, and extensor surfaces, may occur in connection with obesity.
- Hirsutism in women may result from increased production of testosterone, which is often associated with visceral obesity.
- As discussed above, obesity also cause lymphedema, swelling and neuropathy which can lead to "cold sensation", and other uncomfortable sensation like pain and numbness.

Is there any body part not negatively affected by obesity?

I do not know of any. I did not mention vision changes above. We know obesity causes vision loss. Obesity has higher rates of all sorts of eye diseases like glaucoma, cataracts, and macular degeneration which can cause blindness. Obesity can cause hypertension and diabetes and make them hard to control. These conditions can cause vision loss directly or by stroke. Obesity also cause hearing loss. Hearing depends on the three hearing organelles. They also need good nutrition and oxygen to work properly. Obesity causes malnutrition and damaged blood supplies to these body parts.

Chapter 2. Decision

Why do you put "decision" as your first chapter?

You might say it is obvious that I want to lose weight. This is my decision. I agree that you have made your decision to lose weight. However, for a decision to become a real decision there are so many facets. The decision-making process is actually very complicated. A decision is not a real decision if no action follows. The real decision is always followed by more decisions and actions. In this chapter, we will look into how decisions are made and guide you how to make the right decision and choose right actions to lose weight.

Success is the result of right decisions.

In the process of a weight loss journey, what do you mean "real decision is followed by many more decisions with action?"

A decision means to decide what you want and how you will achieve it.

A decision without more decisions and actions is just a small part of the decision-making process, such as information gathering.

Can you give me an example?

You want to lose weight. This is your decision and goal.
This decision is based on much information. Some you consciously gathered; some you may not be conscious of.

Here are some of the follow-up decisions and actions to take:

- how much weight to lose.
- what measures to take.

- how you can follow through these measures.
- when to get up.
- what exercise to do and how long.
- what to eat or not to eat.
- You might decide to walk to work.
- You might stand more during working time.

What is the decision-making process?

The decision process is actually very complicated. It is comprised of desire, collecting information, and action, and then refining of desire, action and gathering more information.

Desire: what you want
Information: the reason/how to achieve or get it; the feasibility
Action: what you do to achieve it
Collection of more information
Refine your goal
Refine your action
Repeat this process until you achieve your goal or make a new decision and set a new goal

How can you make the correct weight loss decision?

- Be specific, for example, I want to lose 20 lbs in the next six months. This is specific. The more specific the decision, the greater the chance to carry through and the more likely you will succeed.
- Be informed. You need to collect information and sometimes you need to consult a specialist or talk to friends to make a weight loss decision safe and achievable. Weight loss is a complex process. If a wrong decision is made, it can be detrimental to your health and life.
- Take action. Everyone is different. You need to find the right action for you.
- Refine your decision based on your result and experience in the weight loss process. You can refine your decisions on how much to lose and how to do it in the process of weight loss.

What are the pitfalls in weight loss decisions? And how can this book help me?

- Specific goal: We do not want you to set up an unrealistic and unscientific goal for weight loss. I knew a man who wanted to pursue a girl and wanted to lose 30 lbs in a month. He set up a goal which is not healthy and sustainable. Although he achieved his goal by starving, it is not sustainable. Well, he lost his weight as he wanted and got his girl. He ended up in the hospital emergency room for irregular heartbeat and gained all the weight back and more afterwards.

This book will help you set up a scientific goal. We recommend one pound per week for weight loss. For total weight loss, I recommend five units of BMI. For example, if you have a BMI 40, I recommend getting your BMI to 35 as your first achievable goal. Please refer to Chapter 1 if you want to know more about what BMI is and how we calculate BMI.

- Information. These days we have too much information about almost everything. If you want to buy a weight loss book, you have hundreds of different titles from which to choose. We call it information overload. When we have information overload, we lose the ability to make the right decision and risk making a wrong decision.

This book provides core information for you to make the best decision and sometimes, we provide the decision and solution for you. We will recommend "forming a habit" to reduce your decision-making process. You can have more energy working on your action to lose weight.

- Action is very important to achieve your goal. Achieving your weight loss target is like everything else. Every day, you can do or not do something. The dos and don'ts form your successes. This book provides both evidence and experience-based recommendations for you. Some recommendations might work for you, some may not. This is like a toolbox from which you can choose.

What is special about the decision-making process for weight loss?

- Obesity is a disease. You are battling a disease. You need a professional to help you. At the same time, you also need determination to follow through.
- Some decisions professionals need to make for you, like which medications to take or not to take. You need professionals to make

sure you do not have other conditions like Cushing's disease or hypothyroidism.

- Some decisions you need to make yourself like moment to moment decisions: to stand or to sit, to exercise or rest, have something to eat or not to eat, what to eat, how much to eat.
- Ultimately you are the decision maker, but weight loss is very complicated. There is so much information, and everyone has an opinion, e.g., a diet might be working for you, but not working for her. Everyone is different. The specific cause for obesity is different, therefore you need to work with a professional to find out the actual cause for your obesity.

Chapter 3. Determination and Motivation

Will it be easy to follow your way of losing weight?

Weight loss is not easy. You have to work on it. You have to pay attention to it every meal, every day. Even if you have formed a healthy lifestyle, you are still facing many decisions, lots of temptations, and challenges. If your weight loss comes easy, you really need to talk to your doctor to make sure you do not have something bad going on in your body.

How do I get motivated?

This is very personal. You are reading this book. You have your motivation. Here are a few examples.

- Olivia is a 45-year-old woman She has been tired of being tired. She wants to enjoy her life more.
- Cora, 46 years old is expecting her first granddaughter. She was so heavy that she was not able to walk a few flights of stairs without getting out of breath. She wants to help her daughter and see her granddaughter go to college.
- Amelia, 35 years old, has never enjoyed sex. Now she is in a new relationship. She is afraid of taking off her clothes in front of her partner. She wants to change that.
- Henry, a 65-year-old engineer, just retired and wants to travel to see the world.
- Tom, a 44-year-old, takes four diabetes medications, four blood pressure medications and one cholesterol medication. He wants to change that.
- Luna, a 38-year-old mom, was not able to help her son practice riding a bike since she cannot run a few yards. She felt ashamed. She wants to change that, so she can help her children.

- Jack, a 48-year-old school teacher, has not had energy and libido for many years. He is also developing diabetes and fatty liver. He wants his life to be better.
- Ben, a 72-year-old retired software engineer, is taking more than 300 units of insulin every day, but his sugar still cannot be controlled.
- …

I was motivated and then I lost motivation. How can I stay motivated?

It is hard to keep motivated all the time. Here are a few things you can do to keep yourself motivated.

- Make a promise to yourself whatever it may be and make yourself accountable. Oliva is expecting her first granddaughter. She wants to be there for her. She put a picture of her daughter and then her newborn granddaughter on her refrigerator. Whenever she sees the picture, it reminds her of her promise and keeps her motivated.
- Tell your friends and family your goal and how you are going to reach it. Tell them your progress. Luna told her story on facebook and she made the promise to all her family and friends to keep updating her progress every week.
- Asher made a promise to his doctor and visits his doctor every two months. When the appointment comes closer, his motivation is stronger. He wants to show and tell his doctor how much progress he has made, and his doctor always cheers for him.
- Ophelia lost 45 pounds and she wants to keep going and wants to lose another 45 pounds. However, it become harder and harder. She joined a running team. She has been traveling around the world to run. Her teammates are there to cheer her and give her strength to keep going.
- I think it is really a good idea to join an online or offline social group. If there is no group, you can start a group.

What is your motivation and what is the most sustainable motivation in your patients?

I exercise every day. I have lots of patients who ask me how I keep myself motivated all the time. Here is my motivation. Patients come to me to seek advice for healthy living every day. If I cannot do it, how can I expect my patients to do it? I have some days that I feel down, lazy, too cold, too hot. I want to skip. At this time, I have a voice saying to myself. At this moment, a patient appears in front of me, asking my advice on how to keep motivated and not giving excuses. Persistence is the only way to succeed.

I also sent out a survey to my patients who have lost 20% of their body weight and kept it off more than two years.

One of the overwhelming answers is that they want to see their children, grandchildren, great grandchildren grow up. Every time, when they feel tempted by "bad food" or an excuse to not exercise, I ask them to picture in their mind that their children, or grandchildren, or great grandchildren come to them to ask advice what they can do at this moment to stay motivated and resist the temptation and do the things they are supposed to do. People found this really powerful. I recommend everyone do it.

Chapter 4. Eat Better-Starts Here

What are the "low-hanging fruit" for eating better?

Low-hanging fruit are those you can pick up without lots of effects. The weight loss process is very complicated and challenging. I always believe that a complicated problem has a simple solution. Low-level fruit for weight loss is those "fattening foods" you need to eliminate or reduce portions. Some are obvious but some are not.

In my practice, I sit down and help my patients pick those low-hanging fruit that have great impact. I have a lady who stopped drinking regular soda and she lost 40 lbs simply by doing that.

How to identify the "low-hanging fruit" for eating better?

Some are easy to identify. Everyone knows eating pizza which is high fat, high salt and high carbs packs high dense calories.

Some are more difficult to identify. I recommend my patients to keep a food journal so we can sit down and look at it together.

What are the top ten foods to avoid?

1. Pizza. Everyone loves it. I love it. When I first came to America in the 1990s, there was no pizza in China. I thought I should go back to China to open a pizzeria. It smells so good and tastes so good. If I opened a pizza business in China, I definitely would have become a billionaire. However, I am glad I did not. Otherwise, I would be guilt in contributing to Chinese obesity/diabetes epidemic. Now pizzerias are all over China not because of me, and so are obese people and diabetics. 50% of adults in China have prediabetes reported in recent scientific medical journal. Pizza, as we know, just tastes so good because it has high salt, high fat and high carbs. The high carbs release

very slowly and keep your sugar high for a long time. It stimulates your body to secrete insulin for a long time and insulin is the number one fattening hormone in your body.

2. Donuts. What are donuts? They are fried high sugar dough. They taste really good. Again, when I first came to America, we did not have donuts in China. I really love donuts. They taste as good as pizza. Donuts not only have high carbs, but high simple purified sugar. They are not good if not worse.

   Let us look at the nutrition facts of one donut:

   Total calories: 200
   Saturated fat (bad fat): 8g
   Total carbohydrates:22 g
   Refined sugar:11g
   Protein: 2.1 g
   Caffeine: 1 mg

3. Pancakes. These are lots of people's morning favorite. You cannot simply eat one. They come in stacks served with butter and syrup.

If you only eat two of them (you might eat four) with butter and syrups, look at the nutrition facts:

Total calories: 560
Total fat: 14g
Carbohydrates: 90.9
Protein: 8.3 g

Beware, the carbohydrates are refined.

4. Waffles. They are basically the same as pancakes. They have very high carbs and if served with butter and syrup, they have high fat and more carbs. These carbs again are refined carbs. They are really fattening.

5. Muffins. They come in different varieties. They have high refined carbs or added sugar although sometimes you can see something like blueberries, or nuts to make them sound healthy.

Let us look at the nutrition facts of a blueberry muffin (different muffins from different companies may vary):

Calories: 647
Carbohydrates: 68g
Sugar: 39g
Protein: 6 g
Total fat: 19g

You can see a blueberry muffin has lots of sugar and carbs. The blueberries are added to make it be perceived as healthy, but the calories come from carbs.

6. Biscuits with gravy. Many people like this and consider this a comforting breakfast. Biscuits with gravy have high fat and too many carbohydrates.

Let us look at the nutrition facts for one biscuit with gravy. I have seen some people eat two! If this is the case, you need to double the following numbers.

Total calories: 376
Total fat:21g
Total carbohydrates: 34g
Protein:14g

7. Hotdogs and hamburgers. Both of these and other similar food products have packed two bad things into one. Usually they use white bread and processed meat. The processed meats are not just low-quality meat but they are also packed with nitrates. The nitrates are linked to all sorts of cancer. I am an Endocrinologist, but I make diagnoses of all sorts of cancer. The reason is not because I am smart, but because there are just too many of them. We are eating too many cancer-causing chemicals.

8. Anything white, like white rice, white bread, tortilla, naan bread, noodles, pasta. These are refined carbohydrates. They have lost important fibers, vitamins, antioxidants, and other important nutrients. The only thing left is carbs. They digest very rapidly and rush into your bloodstream. The surging blood sugar agitates your pancreas to secrete too much insulin, thus causing reactive hypoglycemia (low sugar). People tend to eat even more.

These days China, Mexico, and India like to consume the above-mentioned carbohydrates and have much higher rates of diabetes. Lots of people do not have increased BMI (body mass index), but they already have developed prediabetes, and a fatty liver.

9. Potatoes. Some people think potatoes are a vegetable. Potatoes are not a vegetable. They are a starch. Starch is a carbohydrate. I am not saying all carbohydrates are bad. What I am saying is that it is bad to mistake potatoes for a vegetable. You might think you are eating something really healthy, while actually just providing carbs. Again, I emphasize here that you need physical activities to match the calories you consume especially from carbs.

The most common ways to prepare potatoes make them even worse. Fried potato chips, French fries, twizzles and patties are loaded with fat. These foods make the high carb into both high carb and high fat.

10. Corn and cornbread. I really hesitate to list corn and cornbread here, since from a nutritional point of view, corn is not a bad choice of carbs. However, research shows consumption of corn is linked to obesity and diabetes. The second reason is that people think this is a vegetable and can eat as much as they want. However, corn is a carbohydrate.

What are the top ten drinks to avoid?

1. Regular soda. I am happy to see the news that regular soda sales have dropped to a 30 year low. People are educated now. They know regular soda has too much sugar. However, some people are telling me that they were drinking 3-5 a day, but now they are only drinking one a day. They thought just one a day cannot be so bad. However, one can of regular soda has 40 grams of sugar. A year has 365 days. 10 years has 3650 days. If you drink one can of regular soda a day, you will consume 146,000 grams which equals 320 lbs. (Hopefully your weight is less than 320 lbs)!

   1 can of soda=40 gram of sugar
   1 can of soda per day for one year=32 pounds
   1 can of soda per day for 10 years=320 pounds

Most recently I saw Laura who was referred to me for uncontrolled diabetes. She was taking concentrated insulin (U 500) over 300 units every day. Her sugar was still over 300s. She claimed that insulin had no effect on her. It turned out that she was drinking regular Pepsi 20 cans a day. This is the most I ever heard! Initially she said there were no way for her to cut down. However, she did. Now she is drinking one a day. Her sugar dropped like a stone. Her insulin dose was cut down to below100 units daily and I was able to take her off concentrated insulin. She was able to lose 20 lbs also. Now she is working to stop the last can of Pepsi.

However, diet soda is not good either. The diet soda has also been linked to obesity and diabetes. Some research reported that the diet soda increases your craving for sweets. Other research reported that diet soda could change our gut bacteria which we now know are very important for our appetite, mood and nutrition. Most sweeteners are chemicals anyway. Some of them are cancer causing agents.

2. Fruit juices, even 100 percent fruit juices. Fruit juices have been linked to diabetes. It has been reported that three cups of fruit juice every week doubles diabetes risk. Fruit juices have too much sugar and make your sugar surge. They raise insulin significantly and cause weight gain. The juices also strip fibers away which have lots of health benefits. Fruit also has very high fructose which needs to be converted in the liver. Some evidence shows that the liver might be receiving too much fructose, get overwhelmed and then develop fatty liver. Fatty liver is a serious condition which can lead to cirrhosis and liver cancer.

3. Sweetened iced tea. If sweetened, do not drink it. It is as bad as regular soda. Some people think it is tea after all. The reality is that sugar is sugar.

4. Energy drinks. Lots of them are marketed to young people. They are not good for you.

They have too much stimulant. For most people, after the stimulant fades away, you may feel more tired than before. Also, energy drinks typically contain high amounts of added sugar, high-fructose corn syrup, and artificial sweeteners. A regular can of energy drink has around 40 g of added sugar which is the same as regular soda.

5. Coffee cocktails, like mocha, cappuccino. They pack in purified sugar and fat which you do not need to lose weight.

6. Milk, even skin milk. It is not good for weight loss. Everybody thinks milk provides the calcium you need. You can get your calcium from lots of other sources without the calories and sugar. Sugar in milk is called lactose. Some people have lactose intolerance and they are even worse. The lactose intolerance can cause your gut to be inflamed and affect absorption of other crucial nutrition.

7. Sweetened non-dairy drinks. I thought soy-milk, and almond milk were better. However, beware, some non-dairy drinks have purified sugar added. I just do not understand why they all have to add sugar into perfectly good drinks.

8. Sports drinks. Most sports drinks are sugar and salt (sodium, potassium) with different portions. If you are not running marathons, you do not need sports drinks. They pack in extra sugar and salt which you do not need to lose weight.

9. Beer. The sale of beer has decreased somewhat, but consumption is still huge. In America, average adult beer consumption is around 100 liters a year. The effect on diabetes is still very controversial. The calories in beer are so much more than people think. A typical 12 oz beer has around 130-160 calories. The light version usually has around 100 calories. If you drink more than one, your calories are multiplied.

10. Wine. When people drink wine, people do not think about calories. They think they are not sugary drinks, so it is okay to drink. That is wrong. The calories in wine are very high.

Apparently different wines have different amount of calories. Based on winefolly.com, 6 oz of the light alcohol white wine has the least calories of 107, with dessert wine at 275. Regular red wine has more than 160 calories per 6 oz. Other wines are in between.

I like everything you said above. How do I start?

Everyone is different. Some are able to stop eating and drinking all the "bad food" I mentioned above just like flipping a switch on and off. However, not everyone can do that. Some felt deprived. I do not want you to feel that way. I want you to understand why those foods are bad for you and why you are gaining weight. The weight gain is not sudden. It is gradual. Your bad habit is not formed overnight. It takes months and years to form it. Now you want to break it and form a new habit. It is okay to take months and years.

Rose always drank a can of soda with her lunch. She had lots of other bad habits-like eating pizza a few times a week, but she started with this simple bad habit first. She changed to drinking unsweetened tea. As you may know, just by doing that, she was able to eliminate more than 32 pounds of sugar pumping into her system every year. This is just from one can of soda a day. In three months, she was able to lose 10 pounds. She is really encouraged and motivated to do more. Now she told me that she wants to cut down eating pizza three times a week to one time a week. Again, I think Rose did the right thing to start on one bad habit, eliminating it.

Is drinking wine good for you?

There is lots of noise about wine drinking. You can see a lot of heart benefit from wine drinking on google and even some research. However, beware since most of this kind of research was supported by the wine industry.

Recently a research paper was published in one of the most reputable medical science journals, *Lancet* about alcohol consumption and risks. They analyzed mortality of 599,912 current drinkers. They found the drinkers have a much higher death rate from all causes and the rate increased with the amount of alcohol consumption with minimal risk increase at 100 g per week. In this report, they are not talking about fatty liver, cirrhosis or pregnant women with drinking issues.

How do I start portion control?

Portion control is crucial. This is even more important than what you eat. I use my 50% rule. Eat half of what you had been eating before. You can start one meal at a time or all the meals. I recommend starting your dinner first, and if you're still not losing weight, then reduce your day time meal by 50%. You do not need to reduce your non starchy vegetables.

How do I know if I have done enough portion control?

If you have one of the following two symptoms, you have done enough portion control for now. After you lose weight, and if you want to lose more weight, you need to control your portions further.

- If you feel cold while others feel hot.
- You are losing weight.

Chapter 5. What Do You Recommend Drinking and How Much Should I Drink?

What do you recommend to drink?

Water is the king. Water is life and it is the best for your body. Why do you need to add all sorts of chemicals?

Plain water should be the choice for everyone, but I have patients who do not like the taste. They need a different taste. Nowadays, as long as you have the money, there is something you can buy.

Can I drink sparkling water (seltzer water)?

Sparkling water is infused with carbon dioxide. Some are naturally occurring, most are man-made. The simple version is to infuse carbon dioxide into water. You can buy a machine to make it at home.

Four concerns I have if you drink it as your main source of hydration.

- First concern: The carbon dioxide makes water acidic which might erode your tooth enamel which cannot regenerate.
- Second concern: Sparkling water has been reported to make irritable bowels worse.
- Third concern: For patients who already retain carbon dioxide. They have bad lung-like COPD - and cannot get rid of carbon dioxide. It is really not a good idea to add more burden to the body.
- Fourth concern: Bubbles make you unable to drink a lot. You might not get enough hydration under certain circumstances.

Can I drink sparkling mineral water?

If you drink naturally occurring sparkling mineral water, it should be no worse than regular sparkling water. If you are drinking man made sparkling mineral water, and if you have been told to stay away from salt, you might need to be more careful. The minerals contain sodium.

Can I drink flavored sparkling water?

Some artificial fruit flavor is added to the sparkling water to make flavored sparkling water. More chemicals are added to the perfect water. However, these fruit flavors are usually pretty benign chemicals. In other words, they may not be too much worse than regular plain sparkling water. Look at the label, if you find words you do not know, the product may not be too good for you.

Can I drink vitamin water?

Now you can buy water with added vitamins. The water-soluble vitamins are added to water to make people think it is healthy. First, for most people these vitamins are not commonly deficient. Some people already take some sort of vitamins. The only benefit is to make expensive urine. Some versions of vitamin water also add sugar to become sugar water. Some versions add sweeteners to make "zero" calories. Read the "sweetener chapter" in my diabetes book for more information.

Can I drink alkaline water?

We use pH to measure the acid-base of a solution. The scale is from 1-14. If it is around 7, we call it neutral; if < 7, we call it acidic; if >7 we call it alkaline.

Pure water is around 7 which is neutral. Most tap water is around 7 or below. Some natural spring water has pH above 7.

A lot of health benefits have been claimed by sellers.

Can I drink tea?

Tea, especially green tea has been suggested to help people lose weight. Other beneficial effects include lowering cholesterol and antioxidant effects. However, many claimed good effects have not been really clinically proven.

Can I drink too much tea?

If you drink real tea, it is pretty safe. However, lots of products are claimed as tea but are not real tea. There are reports that renal failure was linked to drinking "too much tea". Tea is also a stimulant which might cause anxiety, palpitations, insomnia, etc. Therefore, I do not recommend that people drink tea in the afternoon.

Is it a good idea to add fruit like strawberries or cucumbers to the water to add some taste?

This practice is very common in hotels or some meetings. If you like the taste, it is not a bad idea. Citrus fruit, such as lemons, limes, and oranges, are often the water enhancers. Other fruits are also becoming popular. Try crushing fresh raspberries or watermelon into your water or adding strawberry slices. Cucumber and fresh mint are refreshing flavors as well. Remember to wash them well before adding to the water. The water with fruit easily becomes stale. Make sure to only drink if when freshly made.

Can I add stevia to my water?

I think there is no reason you cannot do that.

I do not like the taste of stevia. Do you have any other natural sweetener I can use?

Another very good natural product is monk fruit extract. You can buy it from Walmart. It is not expensive at all.

Can I use sugar-free drink mixes?

There are all kinds of sugar-free drink mixes. There are all kinds of brands. Personally, I do not like the taste and feel unhealthy because they are all chemicals, like aspartame, acesulfame potassium, food colors, and many other. If you won't drink water or the above-mentioned versions, then go ahead and use the product. I do not recommend them because they are really not good for you.

How much should I drink?

It is a simple question but not easy to answer. It depends on your activity, your surroundings (temperature, humidity, etc.), your kidney function, medications and your weight. Most people recommend drinking half an ounce to one ounce of water for every pound of body weight. For example, if you weight 100 lbs, you are recommended to drink 50-100 ounces of water (one oz equals 30 cc).

Can I drink too much water?

Yes, you can. Water intoxication is a very serious condition. People can die from it. However, for most people the kidney has a very large capacity to get rid of excessive water.

Chapter 6. Start with a Good Breakfast

I do not like breakfast. Can I skip it?

I heard that if I do not eat breakfast that my body will go into starvation mode, and I would never lose weight. **It is not true.** I have not seen any scientific evidence. Everyone is different.

Here is the advice I give to my patients.

Sugar is just "cash in your pocket" ready to be spent. Fat is just like savings in your bank. If you have enough cash in your pocket you would not go to your bank to withdraw the savings, this is the same for your body. If you do not have times of fasting, your body does not have opportunity to burn the fat. If you skip your breakfast, if you are not snacking all the time, if you are not feeling sluggish, shaky, or weak, and if you do not feel starved before lunch, then you are okay to skip your breakfast.

All the breakfast foods I am eating are either fat or carbs. How can I change that?

- Most people eat one thing day after day. If you are one of those people, you can start to change one day a week and progress to change every day in a week. This can happen in a month or in a year. It is okay to take longer. As I discussed earlier, the bad habit is formed in years, sometimes it takes years to unwind.
- If you are eating all varieties of "bad breakfast" in my list, you can start to eliminate one by one. Iris replaced her hashbrowns with egg whites and she was able to lose five pounds in two months.

- Gather some better alternatives, so you are prepared to start something new. Lots of bad habits are formed in childhood. We were fed cereal at a young age, and we eat cereal every day in the morning. The habit is formed, and we might believe this is the best breakfast to have or only thing to have. Now I want you to embrace new ideas. Keep telling yourself, it is okay to accept ideas about anything including breakfast.

Can you tell me some good ideas about breakfast?

I have to emphasize that everyone is different. You do not need to force yourself to eat if you do not want to. At the same time, I also encourage you to be open to changes.

I want you to assess your physical activity level during the day. If you are very active, it is okay to incorporate some good carbohydrates in your breakfast. If you are not active at all, you would do better to eliminate all the fat and carbohydrates possible, and even the proteins need to be controlled. If you are a person who just wants to eat more of everything, you must have your an activity level match it. So, the most important thing is to match what you eat to activity.

Here is the list you may choose from:

1. Some cooked vegetables. Why not? The reason you do not eat them is because you have never tried them. There is nothing wrong with eating some vegetables as your breakfast. Cucumbers, squash whatever you can eat. People tend to like "fried stuff" in the morning. Do not do that. It is okay to use a little oil (I like to cook my vegetable with a little meat, see below for more ideas) to sauté.

2. Good fruit and berries, as we discussed in the fruit section. I like blackberries, blueberries, cranberries, strawberries, kiwi, guava, cherries, pears, peaches, cantaloupe—with most of them you still need to practice portion control. Fruit has a lot of fructose and that is sugar. You can eat them whole, or you can make smoothies but do not just drink the fruit juice.

3. Greek yogurt. Some versions of Greek yogurt have too much sugar. You need to look at the label. On top of the yogurt you can add some chia seeds to add some texture to it. Chia seeds also add extra protein

and fiber. You can also try adding some flaxseeds onto your yogurt. Flaxseeds have lots of omega-3 oil and magnesium.

4. Try some beans and lentils to replace animal protein and "refined carbs." There are lots of different ways to prepare beans. They are high in protein and relatively low in carbs. They are good replacements for pure carbs. You can buy or make chickpea hummus to eat with whole wheat bread. Edamame can be consumed at any time of the day.

5. Use whole grains to replace refined carbs. You can try barley or buckwheat. You can just boil them or slow cook them overnight. They have lots of magnesium which might help some people relieve leg cramps. Whole grain rye bread is also a better choice.

6. Oatmeal is often recommended. Overnight oats are a good choice. You can put oats, nuts and some milk in a jar and leave it in the refrigerator overnight. You can eat it in the morning.

7. Oat bran flakes are an alternative if you need a quick and easy breakfast.

8. Cereals are generally not a good idea. Some whole grain cereal is acceptable. However, you need to read the ingredients carefully. Some cereal is labeled as whole grain but then some refined sugar is added.

9. If you buy bread, you need to make sure you buy 100% whole grain bread with no added sugar or honey.

10. Quinoa is also a good choice. It has good protein and fiber. The only thing you need to do is to boil it. Quinoa pasta is also good for dinner.

11. Small amounts of cheese. If you are not picky, you can try some vegetables with cottage cheese in the morning.

12. Eggs. I usually recommend no more than one whole egg a day, but you might eat a few egg whites in a day.

13. Avocado can be added to your variety.

14. You can incorporate some sunflower seeds into your breakfast. Sunflower seeds are saturated fat, so portion control is important.

15. All sorts of nuts are very good for breakfast too.

Can I drink cow's milk?

If you want to lose weight, you want to reduce your calories in the drinks as much as possible. I do not recommend you drink milk. Some people are worried about calcium. Calcium are all over the place. For people who wants to lose weight, I recommend taking over-the-counter calcium with vitamin D supplement instead.

Can I drink some milk substitutes?

If you really want to drink something white in the morning, I would recommend unsweetened almond milk. Please check the label, some almond milk has some sugar added. Look online, you can make almond milk yourself, then there is no preservatives or sugars added for sure. The following is a table comparing the common milk.

	calories	Fat g	Carbs g	Protein 9	%Daily Value of calcium
Skin Milk	80	0	11	8	30
1% Milk	102	2.37	12.18	8.22	28
2% Milk	122	4.81	11.42	8.05	29
Whole Milk	136	7.37	19.25	7.3	26
Almond Milk	30	2.5	1	1	45
Flax Milk	70	3.5		8	30
Oat Milk	120	5	16	3	25
Pea Protein Milk	70	4.5	0	8	45
Soy Milk	110	4.5	9	8	30

Lactose free just does not have lactose which dose not reduce the total carbs.

For above chart, we can see almond milk has lowest calories and carbs. The soy milk is very similar to the 2% milk in terms of three major macronutrients.

If you also have diabetes, almond milk and the pea protein milk make the most sense.

My activity level is very low. What can I eat as my breakfast?

If most of the time you are sitting, you really need to change your lifestyle. You are living too easy. Your later life will be harder. You are gaining weight. You will develop hypertension, diabetes, heart disease, cancer, fatty liver, lots of joint pain, and/or back pain.

One option is to start to do something. Start walking. Do not sit all the time. Pick up anything you can do. Moving around is also making your blood flow to reduce blood clots. Whatever difficulties you have, you can always do something. Please consult a physical therapist if you think you cannot do anything.

You might need to consume just a little of everything with no limits for vegetables. Certainly, how much you eat also depends on how much weight you want to lose.

1. 2-3 egg whites. You can boil or pan fry with a few drops of oil. It is easy and affordable. The egg white does not have fat and carbohydrates at all. They are good high-quality protein. It will not increase your sugar. One large egg white has 3.6 grams of protein (17 calories). You can sauté some vegetables such as spinach, cucumber, tomatoes or whatever vegetables you like.
2. This is my favorite. I am like most people who like to eat but not spend too much time preparing it. This breakfast is very healthy and tastes good and is so easy to prepare. I call it chia seed pudding with walnuts.

   Chia seed pudding with walnuts:
   - 2 tablespoons of chia seeds put into 1 cup of almond milk
   - Put in the refrigerator with loose cover overnight
   - Add 7 walnut halves or other nuts.

This is very healthy and does not need much time to prepare.

Chia seeds are very healthy. They are very low in carbohydrates and very high in dietary fibers and protein.

Two tablespoons of chia seeds, roughly 1 oz (28 grams), have: 10.6 grams of dietary fibers (37.6%), and calorie contributing carbohydrates 1.7 grams (6.0%), They have more omega-3 or omega-6 fatty acids than salmon.

3. Roasted vegetables with mozzarella cheese. You can use all sorts of vegetables such as bell peppers, jalapenos, or zucchini, and just add ½ oz mozzarella and roast until vegetables are ready to eat. This is good for cheese lovers. Mozzarella cheese has relatively low fat. Carbohydrates are from vegetables and minimal. If possible, I recommend adding more vegetables.

My level of activity is moderate. I have to walk around during work time. What do you recommend for my breakfast?

If you have some physical activity, you can have many more choices. You can add 15 carbs into your breakfast, like one slice of whole wheat toast and some good fruit like blackberries.

My own activity is low to moderate. Every day, I go to the gym for exercise for 30-45 minutes and I walk from one exam room to another throughout the day.

Here is my breakfast:

- 2 hard-boiled egg whites.
- 2-3 tablespoons prepared oatmeal with some sliced almonds and 3-5 walnuts.

I am not trying to lose weight but maintain my weight. I weigh 138 pounds with shorts on. If you are 200 pounds and trying to lose weight, try my breakfast.

The above three breakfasts are still very good for you.

- You can increase your portions.
- You can add one piece of whole wheat toast.
- You can add one low fat yogurt.

- If your blood pressure is not high, you can add one or two pieces of bacon (has lots of salt). The reason I am okay with my patients eating bacon is that it has its own portion control. I am not expecting you to eat more than two pieces. One piece is around 10-12 grams.
- If you really like traditional fruit, you can add half an apple, or half an banana. Do not eat both.
- You can eat a whole kiwi, or a whole plum, or a whole small peach.

I am a manual laborer. What can I eat?

If you have very strenuous work or exercise or training all day long and you are still gaining unwanted weight. I still do not recommend eating a traditional breakfast like pancakes, donuts, hash browns, or sausages.

Some Asians like to eat rice, noodles, buns, fried dough, or dumplings for breakfast. They are as bad as donuts. They have too many refined carbohydrates.

You certainly need to cut down your portions. Otherwise, you are okay with your breakfast. You might need to eat better for dinner.

Chapter 7. What Can I Eat for Lunch/Dinner?

Can I skip lunch/dinner?

I have patients ask this question. This a simple question, but the answer can be complicated. My answer is- it depends.

If your activity level is very low. You do not need to eat a lot. Whatever you are eating, you are eating too much now since you are not losing weight. You can skip your lunch, but do not overeat at dinner and go to bed soon after.

I have patients who skip a meal and eat large portions the next meal. Especially it is not a good idea to eat a large dinner. The food stays in your stomach and stimulates insulin all night and so you gain weight.

What can I eat for lunch/dinner?

I think you can eat anything. The idea is that you need to cut down on meat and carbs. The amount you eat needs to match your activity level. Portion control is the key.

What are the main ingredients for lunch/dinner?

Vegetables should be the main ingredients.
You can add a small amount of real meat (not processed), shrimp or fish.
You can add some carbs which include fruit. Do not eat fruit as snacks. I do not recommend snacking.
You can add some healthy oil like avocado or olive oil.

Again, the main ingredients of your healthy lunch should be

- A lot of vegetables, raw or cooked. I recommend you eat one pound, distributed to three meals a day. Starchy vegetables are not the vegetables talked about here. All variety of mushrooms are recommended.
- Small amounts of real meat, fish, shrimp, or cheese
- Appropriate amounts of good carbs (whole grain)-depending on your activity level

What are the vegetables you recommend?

amaranth greens (Chinese spinach)	greens (collard, kale, mustard, turnip)
artichoke	hearts of palm
artichoke hearts	jicama (Mexican turnips)
asparagus	kohlrabi (German cabbage)
baby corn	leeks
bamboo shoots	mushrooms
beans (green, wax, Italian)	okra
bean sprouts	onions
Beets (not sugar beets)	pea pods
Brussels sprouts	peppers
broccoli	radishes
cabbage	rutabaga

bok choy (Chinese cabbage)	salad greens (chicory, endive, escarole, lettuce, romaine, spinach, arugula, radicchio, watercress)
carrots	sprouts
cauliflower	squash (cushaw, summer, crookneck, spaghetti, zucchini)
celery	sugar snap peas
chayote squash	Swiss chard
coleslaw (packaged, no dressing)	tomatoes
cucumbers	turnips
daikon (Chinese radish)	water chestnuts
eggplant	yard-long beans

What are the starchy vegetables, and do I need to have portion control?

The starchy vegetables have relatively high non-fiber carbs. Here are the common examples: corn, plantain (potatoes, yams, sweet potatoes), taro, green peas, winter squash (such as acorn, butternut squash), parsnips.

I recommend you have good portion control for corn, plantain, taro, parsnip. You need to cut down other carbs if you eat these starchy vegetables. Carrots have some starch and sugar also. Beets have some carbs also. Comparing to potatoes, beets have much less carbs but more other nutritions. I do not worry about them too much. Although they have relatively high carbs, they have high fibers also.

My activity is very low. What is your recommendation for me?

Again, it is very important for you to make some changes in your activity level.

I recommend you eat 20 g of carbs or less.

You can choose from the following fruit:

- 1 medium apple
- 1 medium peach
- 1 medium plum
- 1 medium orange
- 2-3 small mandarins/tangerines
- 1 medium kiwi
- 1 medium persimmon
- 1 small banana/half of large banana
- 100 g of grapes
- 100 g of blueberries/blackberries/strawberries
- 100 g of figs

You can also try

- 1 piece of whole grain (wheat or barley) bread.
- Half cup of buckwheat
- Half cup of bulgur
- Half cup of quinoa
- Half cup of brown rice
- Half cup of pasta or rice
- Half cup of various beans
- Half cup of sweet potato

My activity is moderate. What is your recommendation for me?

Examples of moderate activity are: you are standing all the time, you go upstairs and downstairs frequently, you do some moderate exercise.

You can eat 40 grams of carbs (you can double the above items) and 3 oz of meat or fish.

I am a manual laborer. What is your recommendation for me?

If you are a construction worker, or athlete, or mover, you can have 60 g of carbs and 4 oz of meat or fish. The numbers here are not really important. If you are gaining weight or not losing weight, it means you are eating too much in comparison to your level of activity (metabolism). You need to cut your consumption. My usual recommendation is to reduce your portion by half.

You can triple the portion of above carbs.

Again, do not snack.

Do you have special recommendations for dinner/supper?

- Do not eat dinner too late.
- Prepare some soup to fill your stomach.
- Do not snack before bed.
- Eat more vegetables and cook them if possible

What are your favorite foods, and how do you prepare them?

The following is my everyday food. You can see they are all natural and not processed (part of nutrient has been stripped or mixed with low value carbs or fat or other chemicals). They are low carbs and low meat recipes. Also, they are easy and good for one or two persons. I have lots of patients and they live by themselves and feel that cooking for one person is too much trouble. You can do good things for yourself. You do not just do them for other people. Another reason I wrote this section is because I want to introduce some really good food for you to lose weight and with a simple easy recipe/idea.

Asparagus

Asparagus is my number one favorite. When I am home alone, this is the one dish I go to. It is so easy to prepare. I sometimes grill, bake, or just pan-fry it. In reality, I do pan-fry more often. I just cut off the dry ends, and then rinse them. I add some vegetable oil in the pan to grease the pan, add a little water, put in the asparagus, put it on the stove and turn on the heat. After you see the steam coming out of the pan, you just stir a few times until it is dry (do not add too much water—otherwise it will never dry). That is it.

I also make asparagus chicken stir fry.

I use 4 oz of chicken breast cut into small pieces. I marinate it with some cooking wine, salt, and add some black pepper or any seasonings you like. I just wait a few minutes. If I am in rush, I do not even wait and stir fry using a prewarmed pan with a teaspoon of vegetable oil.

Just add the precooked asparagus and chicken together. You have an asparagus chicken stir fry.

You can add more vegetables in the dish - like cooked carrots (again, carrots have lots carbs, but I do not worry about it).

You can use different meats or peeled shrimp.

Celery

My second favorite is celery. Most of the time, I just boil it until it soft, and then I add some soy sauce. Sometimes, I cook it with tofu. I boil celery and cook my tofu separately. Then I mix them together with some olive oil. You can add some black pepper or any other spices if you like.

Carrots and daikon soup

My third favorite is carrots and daikon soup. American soup is mostly cream based, or broth based. It either has too much salt or too much fat. This soup is good. It does not have fat, and it does not have too much salt. You just cut some daikon and carrots into cubes, add a few dried shrimp (you can buy them from an Asian grocery store), add an appropriate amount of water and boil until soft. You can eat this before your meal to curb your appetite. This soup has low calories. You can also use it as a snack (I do not recommend snacks over 10 g of carbohydrates or 50 calories).

Raw Jerusalem Artichoke

It is very easy to prepare. Just rinse well. Cut into thin pieces. Sprinkle with salt and wait for 10 minutes. Then you can enjoy with whatever sauce you like.

Spinach

Another of my favorites is spinach. I eat it by itself or with bean sprouts. You can eat it raw, but I prefer to stir-fry it with a few drops of vegetable oil

Dandelion leaf

You can eat raw, or cooked. I just add it into salad or cook the same as spinach.

Zucchini

There is nothing easier than cooking zucchini. You can cut zucchini into whatever shape you like. Just stir-fry. It is also easy to grill.

Bok Choy

This vegetable sounds like Chinese. You certainly can buy it from an Asian store. You should try it at a Chinese restaurant to see if you like it.

I cook it with a lot of garlic and ginger. It is so easy and tastes really good.

Here is what I do.
-Wash bok choy very well. You do not want to eat dirt. I usually cook one pound.
-Wash some mushrooms (whatever kind as long as edible).
-Prepare some garlic (I use a lot)- you can mince them or just chop them. Certainly, you need to peel.
-Prepare some ginger. You can just cut into pieces or grate it if you like. You do not have to add it if you do not like ginger.
-Use a saucepan, add 1 teaspoon of vegetable oil and then add your prepared garlic, ginger and mushrooms. Last add in the bok choy. I also add a little water (like half a cup).
-Turn heat to high and raise it to a boil for 3-5 minutes until it becomes tender.
-It is ready to serve!

Chicory

It is really nutritious. It has lots of fiber and has been shown to reduce triglycerides and cholesterol. You can eat as other vegetables like bok choy and lettuce.

Chicken broccoli

You might have been to a Chinese restaurant and had chicken broccoli. I usually use chicken breasts which are easy to handle. I cook the broccoli and chicken breasts separately. I just cut the chicken into small pieces. Then, I add some chicken seasoning with garlic. It just takes a few minutes to cook the chicken. I cut the broccoli into pieces, and just boil them until they are a little soft (not too long, otherwise, it will be too soft). Then, I just mix them. You can add salt if you want.

Mushrooms

I really like mushrooms. I eat them raw, or cooked. They have very few calories and carbs. I really do not count the calories in mushrooms. They have plenty of riboflavin, niacin, copper, potassium, and pantothenate.

You can add into salads or mix with all sorts of vegetables or soups.

Chicken salad

I just chop some celery (2 stalks), half an onion and mix them with something else like tomatoes. I also add some different nuts 10-20 pieces (whatever I have like almonds). Use some white or black pepper or whatever seasoning you like. Lastly, I add a few strips of pre-cooked chicken strips. You can also use on a low carb diet.

Onions and mushrooms

I use whatever onions I have and cut them into pieces. Stir fry the onions until soft, then add the pieces of mushrooms and stir fry for one or two more minutes.

Okra

I love okra. It is so easy to cook. You can stir fry it with minimal oil, or you can just boil it or grill it. You can also bake it to make vegetable chips.

Leeks and scrambled eggs

Leeks have lots of good fiber and prebiotics. I really love them. They are very simple to prepare. Wash the leeks and cut into one-inch long pieces. Make the scrambled eggs first and take them out. Leeks only need to cook a few minutes until it changes its color. Add the precooked eggs. Lightly salt and you can enjoy.

Green beans

They are so easy to prepare, just like okra. You can boil them. I like to stir fry or grill them.

Baked or steamed squash such as acorn squash

Acorn squash has lots of vitamins and fiber. It is very easy to cook. I just cut it into pieces, rinse off the seeds and bake or steam it. You can season with anything you like. The carbs are lower than potatoes. I use them to replace my carbs from potatoes, rice or bread. Remember it is also starchy. You need portion control.

Caprese salad

This is a simple Italian salad, made of sliced fresh mozzarella, tomatoes, and sweet basil, seasoned with salt and olive oil. It is low in carbs.

Avocado

Avocado is very popular now. I've tried some avocado dishes and they're not bad. You can add avocado into any salad. I can make a salad with all sorts of greens like spinach, kale, and cucumbers, and add half an avocado. This is a very low carb dish. In all sorts of salads, I like to add some nuts.

You can also make yourself a sandwich with avocado. Vegetarians like to eat this. You can try it using whole grain wheat bread. Use one piece if your activity level is low.

Edamame

Edamame is immature soybeans. One cup of frozen edamame has 3 grams of sugar, but 6 grams of fat, 6 grams of dietary fibers and 12 grams of protein. It also has plenty of iron, calcium, magnesium and potassium. I consider edamame a healthy food.

I roast or boil and then incorporate in salads or other dishes.

I make edamame chicken stir fry.

Depending on your activity and how much you should eat, here is what I do:
4 oz of chicken breast-cut into pieces or strips. Mix with small amount of salt, pepper, any other seasoning you like, and a small amount of cooking wine. Put into a saucepan with small amount of vegetable oil (a teaspoon), stir fry a few minutes until the meat becomes white. I usually remove the chicken and then cook edamame.

-1 cup of frozen edamame. Previously thawed and rinsed. Stir and fry in the same pan we cooked our chicken. Then mix the cooked chicken breast with the edamame.
-Now you can enjoy!

I make all sorts of varieties.
--You can add more vegetables with the edamame if you want. Sometimes, I also add some chopped carrots (orange color), tomatoes, bok choy, or broccoli.
-You can also switch the chicken breast to other meat. I like chicken breast since it is white meat and also very easy to cook. But you can change to any kind of meat or shrimp.

Quinoa

Technically speaking, quinoa is not a grain, but we eat it as a whole grain. It is a seed from the *Chenopodium quinoa* plant. It is widely cultivated in South America.

These days I do not eat white rice. When compared to brown rice, quinoa is much healthier.

Look at the nutrition facts for one cup of cooked quinoa and one cup cooked brown rice from nutrionfacts.com

	Quinoa	Brown Rice
Calories	222	200
Protein(g)	8	4
Dietary fiber(g)	5	3
Non fiber carbs (g)	34	40
Fat(g)	3.6	3

It also has eight complete essential amino acids for humans (the building blocks of protein).

Quinoa also has more minerals and vitamins compared to rice. I use quinoa as a substitute for rice. It is also gluten free if you are on a gluten free diet.

I like the crunchy and nutty texture.

The main way to cook quinoa is boiling.

Here is how I use quinoa:

Black bean veggie quinoa
-Prepare your vegetables- I like celery and carrots- chop them into the size you like and stir fry a few minutes with a teaspoon of vegetable oil.
-Stir in your rinsed quinoa (one cup) and black beans (need to be precooked or canned-the amount you want), add water to cover. Raise to boil and simmer for 10-12 minutes.
-If you like meat, you can add a few strips - 2 oz of precooked meat or shrimp. (I usually have some precooked meat and store it in the freezer).

I sometimes add mushrooms. Use your imagination! Create a dish yourself!

Tofu
Most Americans know what tofu is but not so many Americans are brave enough to try it. Tofu is really healthy and can help you lose weight. It has very low carbs and high protein. It has many minerals like calcium (so much more than milk), iron, manganese, magnesium, selenium, phosphorus, and various vitamins.

There are more than 100 kinds of tofu and more than 100 ways to eat it. Google it and find the kind and recipe you like and the way to eat it.

Lots of food you will like after you are used to it. Try some tofu at a Chinese restaurant and then you can try to cook it at home.

I like to use tofu to make soup (see below).

Soups

Warm soups help soothe your stomach and adjust your appetite. If you have no appetite, soup can stimulate it. If you feel hungry all the time, it can quench the hunger.

Tofu soup
You can use any kind of tofu to make soup. Basically, you add tofu into water and boil it. Certainly, you want to add some seasoning to raise the taste. You

can try adding anything you want into the soup. You can add the below soup (tomato egg soup). You can add some basil to make tofu basil soup. You can add some shrimp to make tofu shrimp soup. If you want to have a little meat taste, you can add some meat. You can incorporate tofu very easily to your recipe.

Tomato egg soup

Nothing is easier to cook than this soup. You just cut a tomato, put it into boiled water until it boils again. Then add a beaten egg and stir a few times with a spoon. Add whatever seasoning you like. This soup is good to curb your appetite.

Duck (Chicken) bamboo shoot soup

I love this soup, and it is easy to make. The only challenge for you is that you need to go to an Asian store to buy bamboo shoots-whatever kind they have. If fresh it is good. If it is dried, you need to soak them first and rinse them well. The carbohydrates are very low in this soup so you can use it in a low carb diet.

You need to use a slow cooker. Put in the following ingredients. You can make any variety.

- One half duck (you can use the breast only), or if you do not like duck, you can use chicken. You can cut into pieces or not.
- Add some cooking wine, ginger or anything you add when you cook duck or chicken.
- Add some black fungus (wood ear or cloud ear mushrooms). If you do not have black fungus, you can try any other mushrooms
- Bamboo shoots. Cut into small pieces.
- Add two pieces of precooked bacon.
- Add water to cover everything.
- Add appropriate amount of salt depending on how many ingredients you have. Less is okay. Then you can adjust when you eat it later.
- Slow cook overnight.

You can use lotus roots to replace bamboo shoots or add both if you have them. Beware, lotus roots have more carbs.

Enoki Egg Soup

This is another good soup to try. It has very low calories, and low carbs. You might ask what is enoki. This is a kind of mushroom. As a matter of fact, you can use any kind. I want to expand your food variety. Google it. You can buy fresh or dried. You even can buy from Walmart.

If you, like me, like ginger and green onion, you can do the following, otherwise, use any herbs or seasoning you like.

If you use the dried enoki, I recommend presoaking a few hours, but you do not have to.

- Use a teaspoon of vegetable oil, raise the temperature a little and add grated or sliced ginger and pre-cut green onion and stir a few times.
- Add prewashed enoki- 1-2 oz depending on how much you want to eat. Again, it has very low calories and carbs. I do not even count them.
- Add water to cover. If you want fewer solid ingredients, just add more water. Bring to boil. If you use the dried enoki, you might want to simmer for a few minutes until the enoki is hydrated and expands.
- Add beaten egg and stir. I just use one. If you eat eggs often, do not use the whole egg, just the egg white.
- Get ready to enjoy!

Chapter 8. Popular Diets

What is the ketogenic diet keto diet?

Keto diet, short for ketogenic diet, is an extremely low carbs or no carbs diet and high fat diet. The carbs need to be less than 20-45 carbs daily. When we consume such low carbs diet, our body is forced to breakdown fat for energy. The breakdown of fat is to produce ketone bodies. This process is called ketogenesis.

What are the variants of keto diet?

- Standard ketogenic diet (SKD): It typically contains 75% fat, 20% protein and only 5% carbs.
- Cyclical ketogenic diet (CKD): the standard ketogenic diet is very hard for most people long term. So some people created this cyclical ketogenic diet to make it possible. This diet involves periods of higher-carb refeeds, such as five ketogenic days followed by two high-carb days.
- Targeted ketogenic diet (TKD): This diet allows you to add carbs around workouts. It certainly reduces the weight loss, since your body starts to burn carbs instead of fat. It does make it more tolerable.
- High-protein ketogenic diet: This is similar to a standard ketogenic diet but includes more protein. The ratio is often 60% fat, 35% protein and 5% carbs. The protein interferes with the process of ketogenesis, so the effectiveness also is reduced.

Is it true that a ketogenic diet has other health benefits?

The ketogenic diet was first introduced to treat child epilepsy and was reported to be as effective as medication. There are other reports for slowing the progress of Alzheimer's disease, depression and other psychogenic conditions. However, all of these claims have not been confirmed.

What do you need to know before you start the keto diet?

I want you to know the following before you start the keto diet. I recommend you see your doctor and discuss it before you start.

- The long-term weight loss effect is not clear. Most people cannot stay on it long term. Any extreme diet is very hard to stay long term. I consider the keto diet an extreme diet.
- The long-term health effect is not known. The keto diet consumes a lot of meat, saturated fat and cholesterol. All of these have been shown to increase the risk for cardiovascular disease including heart attack and stroke.
- Long term on the keto diet might cause some vitamin deficiency.
- It might change your mood. The effects on mood are varied.
- If you have type 1 diabetes, I do not recommend it.
- If you are taking an SGLT2 antagonist for type 2 diabetes, you need to be careful.
- If you are taking an SGLT2 antagonist for type 2 diabetes with severe pancreas dysfunction, I do not recommend it.
- If you have type 1 diabetes and take an SGLT2 antagonist, you really should not stay on the keto diet.
- If you have moderate to severe liver dysfunction, I do not recommend it. Keto diet increases the burden of liver.
- If you have moderate to severe kidney dysfunction, I do not recommend it, since keto diet increases the burden of kidney.
- If you have gastroparesis, I do not recommend it since the keto diet has too much fat and can make your gastroparesis so much worse.
- If you have significant pancreatic deficiency (history of severe pancreatitis), I do not recommend it.
- You need to monitor your blood pressure carefully since the keto diet might cause your blood pressure to drop too much.
- You need to monitor your blood sugar more closely since the keto diet might cause your sugar to drop too much. You need to adjust your medications. Discuss with your doctor before you start.
- You need to monitor and adjust your diabetes medications since your sugar might drop too much.
- Constipation might be a big problem for you if you already have constipation.
- You will increase your risk for kidney stone if you eat too much meat.
- You will have increased risk for gout if you eat too much meat.

Who are the people you recommend starting the keto diet?

People who are free of the above conditions and who cannot follow my low carb, low meat, whole food diet. They are still eating too many carbs and cheat all the time. I let them try the keto diet and they might have a chance to succeed since they are trying harder to restrict their diet and cheat less.

Why does the keto diet work for weight loss in the short term?

Here are the reasons the ketogenic diet is really working in weight loss short term. The long-term weight loss is not very clear.

- People are eating so many carbs. The keto diet eliminates so many carbs and it has a calorie restriction. Like any other calorie restricted diet, it causes weight loss.
- I have people whose diet was so bad (they drank a few 6-packs of soda a day), but now the keto diet eliminates all of that. I have people who just stopped drinking soda and were able to lose 30 lbs.
- The ketogenic diet leads to low insulin. Insulin is the hormone that makes fat. Now the insulin is so low that fat is being broken down and not being made.
- Insulin is also important to maintain the salt and water. The keto diet also helps you lose water. Your water loss is also responsible for your weight loss.
- The ketos are very small, and they are lost in the urine. You lose something as ketones and ketones also drag out some water weight for you in the urine.

What are the usual foods to eliminate for the keto diet?

These are the major food categories you need to omit:

- Alcohol: Due to their carb content, many alcoholic beverages can throw you out of ketosis.
- Sugary drinks and dessert: regular soda, fruit juice, smoothies, cake, ice cream, candy, etc.
- Grains or starches: Wheat-based products, rice, pasta, noodles, cereal, corn, etc.
- Fruit: All fruit, except small portions of berries like blackberries, blueberries.
- Beans or legumes: Peas, kidney beans, lentils, chickpeas, etc.
- Root vegetables and tubers: Potatoes, sweet potatoes, carrots, parsnips, etc.

- Low-fat or diet products: These are highly processed and often high in carbs.
- Some condiments or sauces: These often contain sugar and unhealthy fats.
- Unhealthy fats: Limit your intake of processed vegetable oils, mayonnaise, etc.
- Sugar-free diet foods: These are often high in sugar alcohols, which can affect ketone levels in some cases. These foods also tend to be highly processed.

What foods are generally recommended for the keto diet?

The following food categories are allowed for a ketogenic diet.

- Meat: all kinds of animal meat and poultry, like red meat, steak, ham, sausage, bacon, chicken and turkey.
- Fish: such as salmon, trout, tuna and mackerel.
- Eggs: whole eggs.
- Butter and cream.
- Cheese: Unprocessed cheese (cheddar, goat, cream, blue or mozzarella).
- Nuts and seeds: Almonds, walnuts, flax seeds, pumpkin seeds, chia seeds, etc.
- Healthy oils: Primarily extra virgin olive oil, coconut oil and avocado oil.
- Avocados: Whole avocados or freshly made guacamole.
- Low-carb veggies: Most green veggies, tomatoes, onions, peppers, etc.
- Condiments: You can use salt, pepper and various healthy herbs and spices.

What are the differences between ketosis and ketoacidosis?

Ketosis is the process generating ketone bodies. As we know, ketosis does not occur if you eat enough calories and balanced food. Ketosis occurs if you reduce total calories significantly, or eat extremely few carbs, or work on extended period of strenuous exercise. Ketosis is a way your body releases the stored energy for your body to use in stressful situations like no carbs, extended time of fasting (starvation), energy deficit, or strenuous exercise.

Ketoacidosis generally refers to a lack of insulin or insulin relative deficiency. With ketoacidosis sugar cannot be metabolized. So, the body breaks down large amounts of fat thus generating too many ketone bodies throughout your body, metabolizing and eliminating them through urine. Your blood becomes very acidic. This can be very toxic to your cells. The process also produces significant water loss due to the sugar and ketones dragging out water with them. Patients also develop severe nausea and vomiting. This is one of the most dangerous complications of diabetes. Early diagnosis and treatment are very important, otherwise the patient can die.

Can the keto diet lead to ketoacidosis?

If you do not have diabetes, especially type 1 diabetes, the chance of developing ketoacidosis is very rare. So far, I have not seen a case report of the keto diet leading to ketoacidosis. However, theoretically, it is very possible in patients with severe pancreas dysfunction.

What is the Paleo diet?

The Paleo diet mimics the diet that Paleolithic Age people ate. The Paleolithic Age is the older part of the Stone Age which is the first known human history. It is before the era of agriculture. People were eating from hunting and gathering meat, fruit and berries. They stayed away from grains and beans. The basic idea is that we humans do not have enough time to adapt to the changes agriculture brings us. This is the reason we have all these problems like obesity, diabetes and cardiovascular diseases.

I consider this a variant of a low carb, or the keto diet. It eliminates the major source of carbs-grains and beans.

What do you think about the Paleo diet?

- It is not a bad diet. I have patients who tried it and were able to lose weight at least in the short term.
- The part I think we are missing here is that process of hunting and gathering. We are hunting and gathering in the supermarket not in the jungle. We are lacking the activity/exercise.
- Agriculture is not the problem. The problem is that our eating and activity are not matched. Please read Dr. Colin Campbell's *China Study*. It is a 20-year study conducted with over 6,000 people from 65 rural counties in China in the 1970s. He found Chinese people at that

time had minimal atherosclerotic cardiovascular diseases, and little cancer in comparison to the same era in the United States. Chinese people were eating agriculture-based carbs for sure. However, look at China now. The Chinese have major problems with diabetes, heart attacks, stroke, and cancer. They are just like Americans. Their physical activity and what they eat are not matched. Consumption is way too much in comparison to the activity.

- Therefore, the key here is not just what you eat. It is the correlation of what you eat with your activity level. One day I saw on the web what the Olympic champion swimmer, Michael Phelps, eats. Apparently, what he eats in a day, I need a week to eat. However, this still might be too much for me. I do not think my level of activity in a week equals his training in a day.
- This can be expensive. It requires everything to be organic and natural.
- You might miss some important nutrients from grains or beans. They have many healthy fats, B vitamins, phytochemicals and antioxidants like vitamin E and plenty of minerals like iron, selenium, magnesium, etc.
- As we discussed, the major issue is that we eat too much as a total. Too much meat means too high fat and cholesterol. Too much meat also increases the burden on your liver and kidneys to get rid of byproducts. Patients with liver failure, renal failure or with high uric acid (gout) are not recommended to go on the Paleo diet.

What is the Atkins diet?

The Atkins diet was developed in the 1960s by cardiologist Robert C. Atkins. It has survived for more than half a century. It is very sophisticated now. There is a full special industry based on the Atkins diet. You can buy hundreds of books as well as meal replacement products and there are programs to join that help you monitor your exercise with your food consumption.

Dr. Atkins' idea is that the problem we are facing is from people using carbs to replace fat. This causes obesity and cardiovascular disease.

Therefore, the core of the Atkins diet is another low carb diet, like the keto diet. It allows protein but not a high protein diet. The main food is fat.

As you know, it is very sophisticated. It is separated into four phases:

- **Phase 1: Induction.** In this strict phase, you cut out almost all carbohydrates from your diet. The only carbs allowed are from green vegetables. Fruit is not allowed. Starchy vegetables are not allowed.

  Your foods are animal meat, fish, eggs, and cheese. Fats are encouraged.

- **Phase 2: Balancing.** In this phase, you are allowed to slowly add back in some nutrient-rich carbs, such as more vegetables and berries, nuts, and seeds, as you continue to lose weight. You can start phase 3 if you think you have enough weight loss.

- **Phase 3: Pre-maintenance.** In this phase, you can eat more healthy carbs from fruit, whole grains and some starchy vegetables. You need to go back to stage 2 if you gain back weight or if you want to lose more weight.

- **Phase 4: Lifetime maintenance.** You can stay on the diet.

  Exercise is recommended but not required.

What do you think about the Atkins diet?

- It is very sophisticated, and you can get all the support you want.
- It has been evolving and adapting to current trends.
- I agree that it is a problem when people use too many carbs, especially the refined carbs to replace fat.
- I think the Atkins diet is another diet switch from carb to fat.
- We need to have a balance between what foods we consume and how much we need to move more.
- As we know, using too much fat and meat to replace carbs can have some consequences too.
- There are the same risks as for the keto diet. See above.
- You need to talk to your doctor before you start the Atkins diet.

What is the South Beach Diet?

The South Beach Diet is a commercialized weight loss program. It was created by cardiologist Arthur Agatston in 2003.

It is another modified low carb diet. It is not as restrictive as the keto and Atkins diets, and it also has more protein in its diet.

It uses the glycemic index and glycemic load to determine which carbs you should avoid. The higher the glycemic index the faster and higher your sugar will rise after you eat.

The South Beach Diet also emphasizes healthy fats, dietary fibers and whole food.

The South Beach Diet has three phases:

- **Phase 1- "body reboot".** This two-week phase is designed to eliminate cravings for foods high in sugar and refined starches to jump-start weight loss. You cut out almost all carbohydrates from your diet, including pasta, rice, bread and fruit. You are only allowed to eat the food they send you.

- **Phase 2 - "steady weight loss".** This is a long-term weight-loss phase. You begin adding back some of the foods that were prohibited in phase 1, such as whole-grain breads, whole-wheat pasta, brown rice, fruits and more vegetables. You stay in this phase until you reach your goal weight.

- **Phase 3- "maintenance".** This is a maintenance phase meant to be a healthy way to eat for life. You can eat all types of food in moderation.

What do you think about the South Beach Diet?

- I think it is not a bad choice if you have money and need a structured diet. They sign you up for different diet level meal plans. They send you the food. This eliminates "thinking work".
- May not be affordable for everyone.
- The menu may be limited.
- You may not be losing weight as you wished.

- Since the carbs are not as restricted as with the keto diet and Atkins diets, it is generally safe to try.
- If you are restricted to the food, they ship to you, it might be difficult to stay on it for long.
- In phase one, the carbs have been drastically reduced, if you have diabetes and are on diabetes medications, your medications have to be adjusted, otherwise it might result in severe low sugar (hypoglycemia).

What is the Dukan diet?

The Dukan diet is a low carb, high protein diet created by French general practitioner and nutritionist, Pierre Dukan in 2000.

The centerpiece for the Dukan diet is the following:

- High protein
- Low carbs
- Eat oat bran (dietary fibers)
- Walk 20 minutes a day.

You can buy the book and follow the book yourself or visit their website to get the approved food, or you can get into a support group and pay a monthly fee. They do not sell the food.

It is separated into four phases:

- "Attack" phase (1-10 days): you eat all the lean protein you can handle, plus 1.5 tablespoons of oat bran and at least six cups of water daily.

- "Cruise" phase (which can last several months), you add unlimited amounts of non-starchy veggies every other day, plus an extra half-tablespoon of oat bran.

- "Consolidation" (five days for every pound you've lost), you can have veggies every day, and you can add one piece of fruit, two slices of whole-grain bread, and one serving of hard cheese. During this phase, you can also have one or two servings of starchy foods and one or two "celebration" meals where you can eat whatever you want.
- "Stabilization" (ongoing), is all about maintenance. You can eat whatever you like, except for one day a week when you follow the all-protein rules from the food in the "Attack" phase. In this phase, you

also eat three tablespoons of oat bran a day and walk 20 minutes every day.

What do you think about the Dukan diet?

- The Dukan diet is another low carb extreme diet which for some people is hard to follow.
- I think you can lose weight especially in the short term since it is low carb with some calorie restriction.
- Especially in the attack phase, it is basically a keto diet.
- If you have diabetes, you need to watch your sugar closely since you may have low sugar.
- If you have hypertension and are on blood pressure medications, you need to monitor your blood pressure closely. You might develop low blood pressure which can cause dizziness, fatigue, and falls.
- If you have liver dysfunction, your liver might have difficulty handling all the protein.
- If you have kidney dysfunction, your renal failure might get worse.
- Again, the protein comes with cholesterol and its long-term effect is not clear.
- However, generally this is not a bad diet if you emphasize the vegetables, fibers and exercise.

What is the Whole30 program?

In 30 days, you only eat moderate portions of meat, seafood, and eggs; lots of vegetables; some fruit; plenty of natural fats; and herbs, spices, and seasonings.

You are not allowed to eat:

- **Any food with added sugar, real or artificial.** No maple syrup, honey, agave nectar, coconut sugar, date syrup, stevia, Splenda, Equal, Nutrasweet, xylitol, etc.
- **Any form of alcohol, not even for cooking.** (And ideally, no tobacco products of any sort, either.)
- **Any grains.** This includes (but is not limited to) wheat, rye, barley, oats, corn, rice, millet, bulgur, sorghum, sprouted grains, and all gluten-free pseudo-cereals like quinoa, amaranth, and buckwheat. This also includes all the ways we add wheat, corn, and rice into our foods in the form of bran, germ, starch, and so on. Read your labels.

- **Any legumes.** This includes beans of all kinds (black, red, pinto, navy, white, kidney, lima, fava, etc.), peas, chickpeas, lentils, and peanuts. No peanut butter, either. This also includes all forms of soy – soy sauce, miso, tofu, tempeh, edamame, and all the ways we sneak soy into foods (like lecithin).
- **Dairy products.** This includes cow, goat, or sheep's milk products like milk, cream, cheese, kefir, yogurt, sour cream, ice cream, or frozen yogurt.
- **Carrageenan, MSG, or sulfites.** If these ingredients appear in any form on the label of your processed food or beverage, it's out for the Whole30.
- **Baked goods, junk foods, or treats with "approved" ingredients.** Recreating or buying sweets, treats, and foods-with-no-brakes (even if the ingredients are technically compliant) is totally missing the point of the Whole30.

You can sign up with the Whole30 program, and they will provide an app which will help you plan your meals.

What do you think about the Whole30 program?

- To me, the practice is very similar to Paleo Diet. Both eliminate grains and legumes.
- I agree with most recommendations. We should not eat those cookies, sweets, treats and any food with added sugars.
- The same thing as other low carb diets. The 30-day crash might cause a problem for diabetes patients.
- Whole grains and legumes are healthy foods too. But if you eliminate them for a long term, you might miss the nutrition from them.
- They provide newsletters and apps to help you start. For some patients, this might be helpful.

Chapter 9. Meal Replacement

What is meal replacement?

Use some formulated bar/shakes or combination to replace the meals. Usually it has significant calorie restriction. You can replace one meal or all meals.

Does it work in terms of weight loss?

It works if you can stick to it because it has very low calories. Studies show most people cannot stick to it over one year. After people get off the meal replacement, their weight usually gets back where it was.

Who do you recommend using meal replacement?

- For some personal reasons like attending a wedding if you want to lose weight quickly.
- You already did the best you can for your diet, but still you are not losing weight, or you want to lose more weight. I might recommend one meal replacement.
- You are living a stressful or chaotic life, and you are eating meals very irregularly and cannot control the portion.
- You do not over eat the next meal if you miss a meal.
- It is also very common for patients to be recommended to use meal replacement before weight loss surgery, especially gastric bypass surgery. It has been shown to reduce liver size and complications.

What are the potential side effects to using protein as meal replacement?

I reviewed the marketplace and saw more products trying to use more protein. High protein diets or meal replacement might help weight loss, but these practices are not risk free. Some risks you need to keep in mind:

- High protein diets and high protein supplements have been linked to increased cardiovascular disease (hypertension, coronary artery disease and stroke).
- It is also linked to a few cancers like breast, colon, and prostate cancers.
- Increased urine albumin excretion which is an early indicator of kidney disease.
- Increased renal stones significantly.
- Increased bone loss.
- Some reports describe the contamination of protein supplements leading to death.
- Some productions increase the rate of acne.
- If you eat too much, you can gain weight as other nutrients.
- Too much protein or supplements can also reduce insulin sensitivity which can cause your sugar to increase.

What are the potential side effects of meal replacement in general?

Depending on different products, and your health, a variety of potential side effects might occur:

- Meal replacement causes rapid weight loss. You can have all the side effects of rapid weight loss.
- Allergy might occur to any component of meal replacement. Replacements usually use protein supplements from whey, casein, soy. If you have food allergy, you need to pay more attention to the ingredients.
- Gastrointestinal manifestation: some products can cause diarrhea and discomfort. Constipation is also common.
- I have patients complaining of headache for some unknown reason.
- Electrolyte disturbance. You need to follow up with your doctor if you have full replacement.
- You might feel weak.
- Your blood pressure might drop. You need to talk to your doctor about adjusting your blood pressure medications.

- Your blood sugar might drop. If you have diabetes, you need to talk to your doctor about adjusting your diabetes medication. Certainly, it is very important to check your sugar.
- Renal stone and gall stone risks are increased significantly.

Should I join a medically supervised meal replacement program?

This is a good idea. The medically supervised programs usually have resource to monitor you better for the above potential side effects. You might also be instructed and educated for a better lifestyle.

The drawbacks are very obvious. It is very expensive and also, they might tend to sell you some supplements you really do not need.

Can I just start meal replacement on my own?

I do not recommend it. At least, you need to talk to a doctor who is knowledgeable enough to give you advice or monitor your changes and adjust your medications.

However, if you are otherwise perfectly healthy, you can try just replacing one meal. I recommend replacing your dinner with 200-400 calories and supplemented with non-starchy vegetables. I find this way is relatively safe and can achieve long term weight loss especially for patients who are not able to lose weight on their own portion control.

Can I buy meal replacements from local grocery stores and what should buy?

The simple answer is you can. I reviewed the line of products. They have at least 10 different kinds and how to choose and what to choose is not an easy task.

I consider the total calories, portion size (affects the price), protein contents, carbohydrate contents, vitamins and possibility for allergy and intolerance.

Most people consume more than 2000 calories per day. If you want to lose 1 pound a week, you need to have a calorie deficit of at least 500 calories every day. People are eating at least 700 calories per meal. I want to replace it with

200 calorie meal replacement for one meal at least five days a week, you are going to replace only one meal in a single day.

It is safe to take 1.45g per kg of body weight if you are otherwise healthy. In other words, you are allowed to take 145 gram of protein if you weigh 100 kilograms (~200 pounds). You can have 45 gram of protein every meal if you want to maintain your weight. However now you want to lose weight. Since we are going to reduce calories about 500. I recommend having protein around 20 grams in the meal replacement.

We do not want the meal replacement to have more than 20 gram of carbohydrates in 200 calories. If you weigh less than 200 pounds or want to lose more weight, you can look for a product less than 200 calories. In reality, we overeat whenever we get the opportunity.

1) Ensure Enlive is a product which meets my criteria. I recommend some people use it. It has 350 calories, 20 gram of protein and 20 grams of carbohydrates. I only recommend for those patients who are consume over 1000 calories each meal.
2) If you want to reduce your calories further. You can try Ensure Original or Ensure Original Nutrition Powder. Both products have around 220-240 calories and a good amount of protein and relatively low carbs. I recommend this product for those patient who usually consume 700-800 calories each meal.
3) If you are not losing weight after one month, I recommend you try Abbot's other brand-Glucerna. I recommend Glucerna Hunger Smart Shake. It has 180 calories, 16 g of carbs (6 g of sugar), 15 grams of protein. The regular Glucerna Shake is essentially the same. You can try this product too.
4) You can also try Boost Glucose Control Nutritional Drink. It has 190 calories, 16 grams of protein. It has total carbs 16 grams and 4 of them is sugar which is not high.
5) SlimFast is also a good product to try. They also have some sensible recipes to try. Again, I recommend you replace one meal. Choose the meal that is hardest for you to control. You can use any product based on your preference. Certainly, the lowest calorie as you think you can live on will produce the best result.
6) Certainly, you can buy these products from local grocery stores or online stores. You can also try other products. The key issue is that you do not choose products which have more

than 350 calories and or have too many simple carbs. You certainly need to pay attention to your allergies and sensitivities for specific contents.

7) You are free to use any other produces. I do not get any loyalty from any products mentioned here.

Can I make my own meal replacement?

Some people like to make protein shakes. In reality, the best is to make vegetable smoothie, or just eat non-starchy vegetable only meal. Again, on these meals, you are not supposed to eat fruits, meat etc.

I am still not losing weight. Can I have two or three meal replacements every day?

If you want to do that, I strongly recommend under doctor's supervision. You might have more chance to have side effects and medical situations to deal with.

Will I have micronutrition deficiency if I stay on meal replacement?

Studies show the commercial meal replacements replace the micronutrition adequately. Especially if you replace one or two meals a day, the chance to have micronutrition deficiency is very rare. You really do not need to take extra vitamins or minerals.

I am still hungry when I replace one of my meals. What can I do?

Here are the options.

- You can eat more non-starchy vegetables.
- Drink more water/tea.
- You can try some medications.
- Get yourself very busy.
- Read the chapter "How to Conquer Hunger?"

When do you recommend fasting?

Intermittent fasting is an extreme form of meal replacement. I recommend this in the following situations.

- You are relatively healthy and able to follow up.
- Not able to practice the portion control.
- Not able to lose weight.
- Not able to control sugar despite very high level of using insulin dose (do not start on your own).
- Not able to control triglycerides despite on many medications.
- Not live alone and able to follow directions.

What fasting regimen do you recommend?

I recommend skip one meal or one day. Some people recommend more extended fasting which need more intensive supervision.

Case. Jason 37-year-old male was admitted to hospital for a few times for acute pancreatitis. He has triglycerides over 10,000 (normal below 150). He has been on three medications for his triglycerides, but his level was still above 1000. At last pancreatitis attack, I was consulted in hospital. We implemented the alternative fasting regimen. He has been doing very well. Now he has not been back to hospital for more than one year. His triglycerides are below 140 on many tests. He did not have a recurrent acute pancreatitis attack since then. He also was able to lose 20 pounds also.

- You can drink water or other non-calorie drinks
- It is okay to eat non-starchy vegetables if you prefer. I found it more tolerable for lots people.
- Need to close monitor you blood pressure and sugar and have a plan in case your blood pressure and/or your blood sugar sugars drop.
- I usually recommend "skip at least five meals" a week. Certainly, you can start with one or two meals a week. If you can skip four meals a week, you might be able to reduce your calorie intake by 6000.
- Again, you need more guideline if you fast longer than one day.

Chapter 10. Physical Activity.

I don't have money to join a gym, and I am living in an unsafe neighborhood. I can't even walk outside. What can I do?

Remember, we recommend you increase your physical activity. You can do more house chores, like mopping your floor every day. You can jog in place (your legs can move up and down but not forward). If you can practice Yoga and tai chi, you can do them any place. You can walk to a shopping mall and walk around there. You can do "wall-sitting". The list is endless, the key is to think about anything you can do to keep moving.

What can I do to incorporate more physical activity into my daily living?

Here are some recommendations you can try to incorporate more activity into your specific situations:

- Park your car a distance from the place you want to go
- Use the stairs if possible, instead of elevators.
- Buy a standing desk for your workplace and home.
- Stand in a subway. Be careful, the bus is less safe to do that.
- Walk in the airport if you are waiting for a flight instead of sitting and "killing time" by surfing the internet.

Do I need a physician's okay to have exercise?

If you think you need to be okayed from your doctor, see one. You need to follow your common sense. You should see your doctor, if you have one of the following conditions:

- uncontrolled diabetes;

- severe cardiovascular disease;
- a balance problem;
- uncontrolled blood pressure;
- severe retinopathy;
- severe osteoarthritis.
- any other condition which concerns you.

I am eating less and walking every day. Why am I not losing weight?

Our body has a weight set point. It is not like that if you pour one pound more water into a bucket you will have one more pound of water. If you eat more, your body actually will try to burn more, but it's just not able to burn everything you eat over the set point. So gradually you have a new set point.

When you eat less, your body tries to burn less, and you might still be overeating compared to your metabolism. Walking is a low impact activity. The average calorie expenditure is four calories per minute. You need to spend at least 500 calories every day to have meaningful weight loss. On the condition that your consumption has been reduced to the level your body need to maintain the basic metabolism requirements, then you need to walk 125 minutes (more than two hours) every day to lose weight. If you are still overeating, then two hours walking is not enough.

Should I do exercise before a meal or after a meal?

I recommend you exercise in the morning while fasting. Your body will burn more fat when you exercise and fast simultaneously.

If you are relatively healthy and do not take diabetes medications, you should not develop low sugar. Not all diabetes medications cause low sugar. Please read my diabetes book. If you are taking some diabetes medication like insulin, you might develop low sugar. You need to discuss this with your physician. Again, safety is paramount. You need to follow your common sense, take precaution and your doctor's advice.

Should I have a snack before exercise?

It is not a good idea to have a snack before you exercise. Your body will burn your snack calories instead of the fat in your body. Again, if you have diabetes, you need to monitor your sugar more closely and know how your body will respond to exercise.

Should I run?

I do not have the statistics, but I have so many patients who developed a problem because of running. If you are not overweight or obese, it is really good for you to run to keep your weight down. If you are 50 or 100 lbs over your ideal body weight, you really should not run. Running has too much impact on your joints. It will hurt your joints sooner or later, and then you have to stop exercising.

Walking is okay. Remember, you need to walk double the distance to burn the same calories running can burn. Running not only burns more calories, but also burns more calories after you stop running than walking.

Walking 1 mile = 80-100 calories / 20 mins
Running 1 mile = 160-200 calories/10 mins

You might burn more if your body weight is higher.

What else do you not recommend in the gym?

Weight lifting is another exercise you should avoid. Obese patients usually have back problems to start with. If you are doing weight lifting, sooner or later, your back will act up and you will have an excuse not to exercise at all.

What kind of exercise do you do in the gym?

I go to the gym early morning like 6 am fasting. I do not eat anything before I exercise but I drink water (tea).

Although I do not need to lose weight, I still do my exercise while fasting. I do not do high impact exercise and I do not do the HIIT (see below). Here is what I am doing every day. Again, I am working out to keep my weight not to lose weight. I am 68 inches and 138 lbs. My BMI is 21.

I am not doing high impact exercise and I do not warm up. My whole exercise routine is simply warm up. Be sure, if you are doing high impact exercise, you need to warm up.

- Lat pull-down machine. I am working on my upper back muscles and shoulder muscles. You can also do it with your palm facing you to let your biceps help you make it easier. I usually do 3-4 sets of 12.

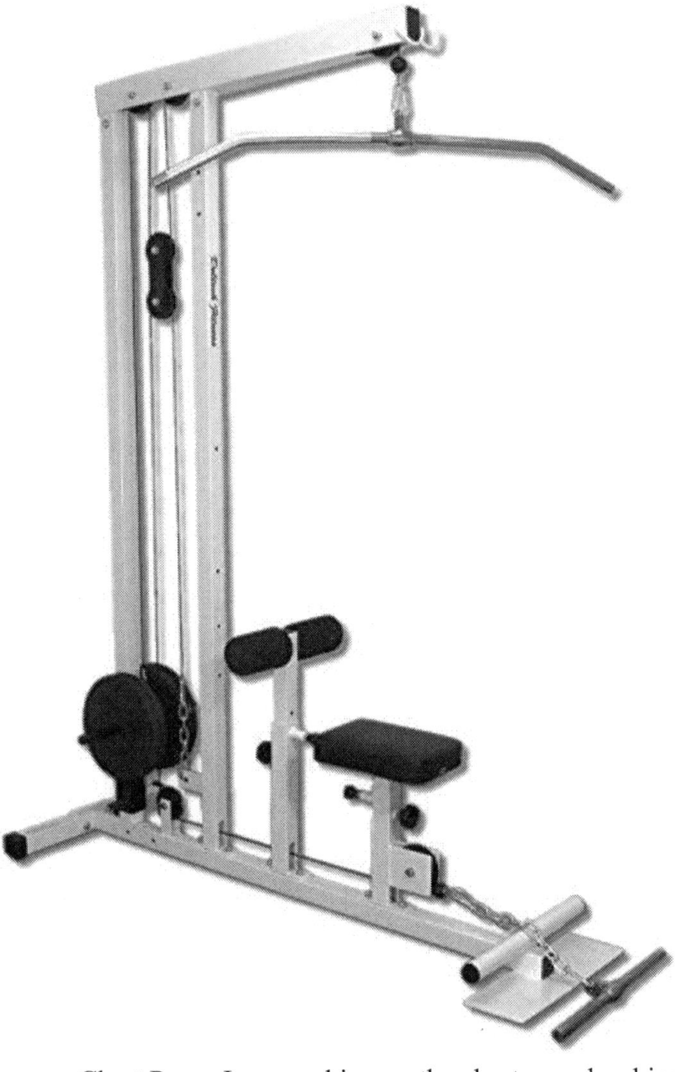

- Chest Press. I am working on the chest muscles, biceps and triceps. I do 3-4 sets of 12. There are all sorts of different chest press machines. I am using the following.

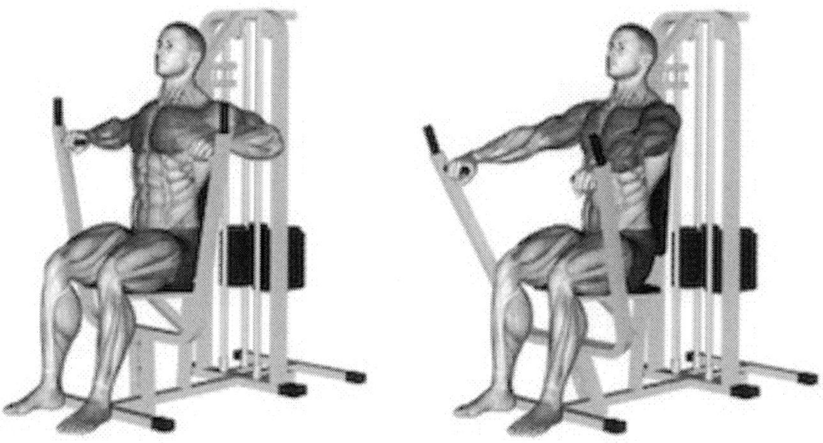

And 3-4 sets of the following Pec Deck Machine for chest muscles and shoulder muscles.

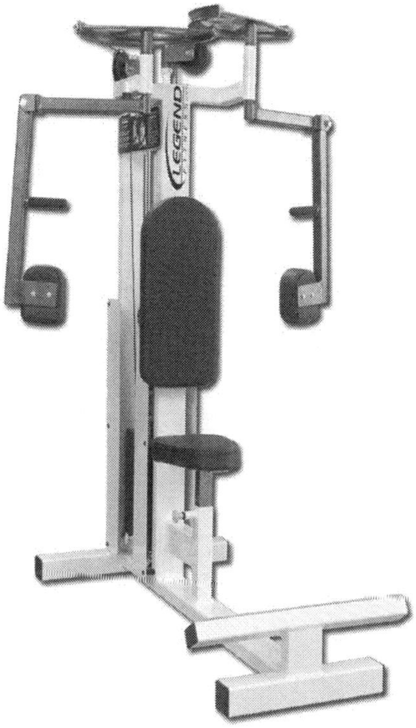

- Then I move to the rowing machine. This machine works out many muscles and does not stress your joints. This is my way of continuing warmup. You can also use this machine to do the High-Intensity Interval Training (HIIT) to lose weight. For HIIT see below.

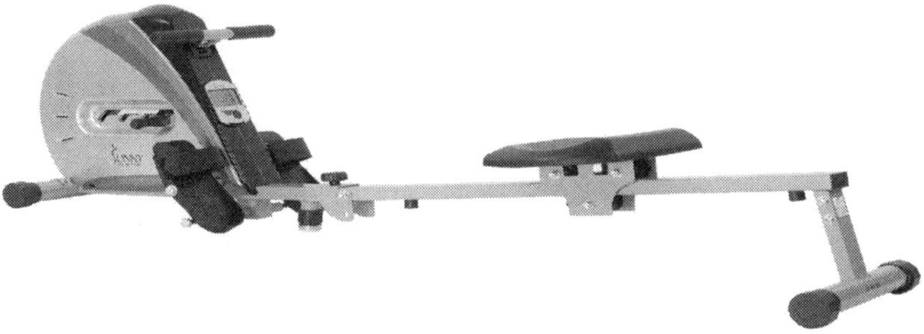

Then I work on both my back and abdominal muscles using back extension and ab bench.

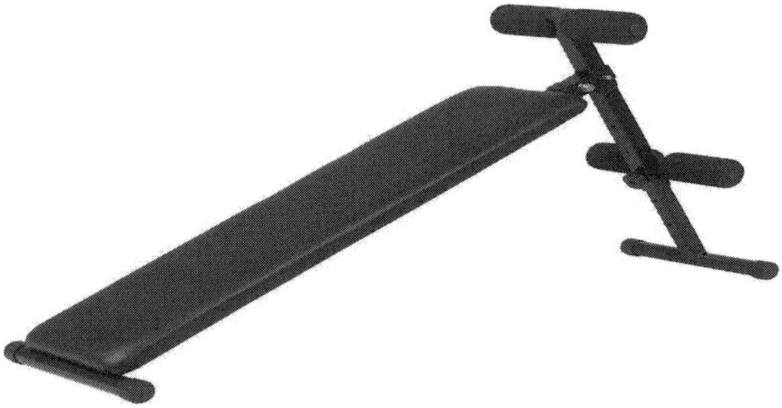

I work out more on the following ab machine.

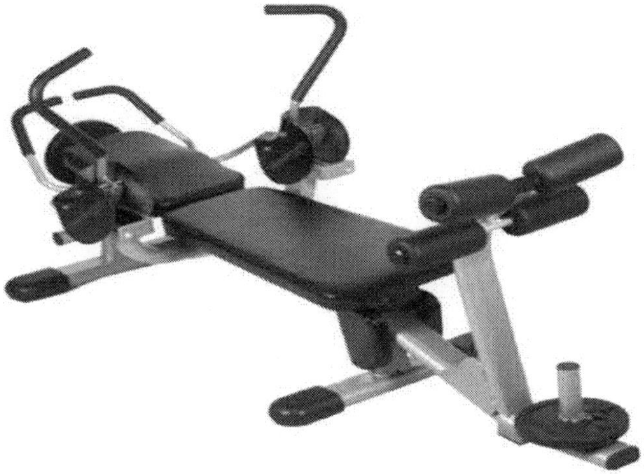

Then I do some pull ups. Now I do up to 15 chin ups and pull ups. Pull ups work both front and back body muscles.

Then I move to the elliptical machine and work on it for 15-20 minutes. The elliptical machine is a stationary exercise **machine** used to simulate stair climbing, walking, or running without causing excessive pressure to the joints, hence decreasing the risk of impact injuries. You can do the high-intensity interval training (HIIT, see the following question) to lose weight.

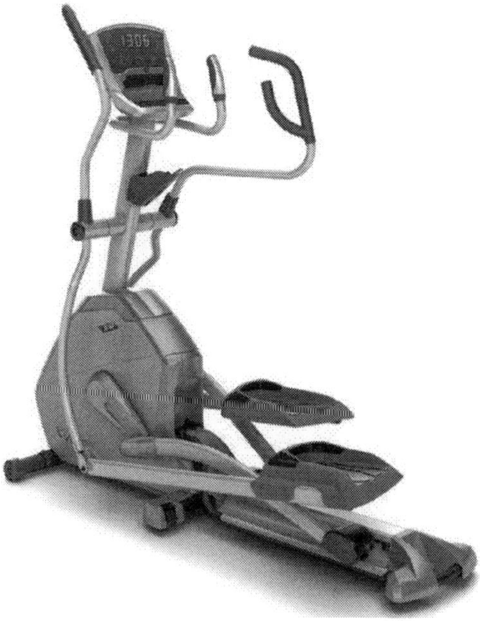

Then I move to the treadmill for 10-15 minutes of running.
Again, I do not recommend my obese patients to run. Treadmill running can lead to foot, knee and even back injuries for obese patients.

At the end, I use the rowing machine or stationary bike to cool down.

Some patients ask why I use so many different machines. Here is my rationale.

- Different machines have different purposes. I want to exercise different muscle groups.
- I never like exercise. I move from one machine to another, so I will not get bored. This is my way to get myself interested and keep doing what I do.
- I won't get tired too quickly.

The pictures of the exercise machines are for illustration only. I do not endorse the particular brand in the illustration. I downloaded the pictures using google with reuse license and I do not have any relationship with the manufactures or sellers.

Is Tai Chi or Yoga good exercise for weight loss?

Both are good exercises and help your balance.

What kind of exercise is the best for weight loss?

High-intensity interval training (HIIT) is the best exercise for weight loss. It refers to an exercise program that is characterized by relatively short bursts of vigorous activity, interspersed by periods of rest or low-intensity exercise for recovery.

It makes sense. You actually need adrenaline to burn the fat. When you have a burst of exercise, your body secretes adrenaline and fat is released for energy. Burst exercise also uses more carbohydrates. The post- exercise energy expenditure is also increased.

HIIT is primarily applied utilizing aerobic exercise, such as running on a treadmill and cycling on an ergometer. Since I do not recommend running, I recommend the rowing machine, or elliptical.

Ideally you should get a personal trainer and start right and gradually. At the beginning, you can do a shorter burst, and more rest.

I do not want to hire a trainer. Can you give me some HIIT workout sheet?

You can google it and find many recommendations.

I looked at this website https://www.self.com/story/a-sweaty-24-minute-cardio-workout-you-can-do-in-your-living-room

What is most important when you advise your patient about exercise?

I use A, B, C to advise my patients for exercise.

A. Acknowledge

- For most people, exercise is boring.
- You need motivation to start but most important you need motivation to continue.
- Exercise is like everything else; you need to start slow and progress slowly. Otherwise you get yourself injured.

Case. I have a 45-year-old patient, Laura. She has been seeing me for hypothyroidism, but recently I also found she had prediabetes. We discussed diet, exercise and lifestyle modifications. She is really motivated, and it happened! A community gym happened to offer three days of free spinning class. She had never exercised before, but she finished her three days of free classes. She was admitted to ICU for acute kidney failure. It turned out that she developed rhabdomyolysis which means that her muscles dissolved and caused kidney failure.

I have so many other patients, who didn't exercise before and suddenly were motivated to exercise. Some hurt their back. Some hurt their knees. Exercise had to stop.

Case: I have Rose who is 65 years old who is seeing me for diabetes. She also has osteopenia which is not bad enough to give her medication yet besides vitamin D and calcium. She heard that Yoga is good for balance. Her gym happened to offer new classes. She joined and really liked it. However, most recently when I saw her she was really down, and had gained a lot of weight. She really surprised me when I saw her. She reported to have an acute spine (vertebral) compression fraction which was caused by Yoga. Rose's case tells us that any exercise is good if you do it properly and gradually. Sometimes even the activity you did before, if you stop it for a while, you need to build it back up gradually. Injury can really cause you a lot emotionally and physically. I recommend people to exercise, but safety is paramount. A qualified personal trainer is really helpful, although I saw a too zealous personal trainer before. In Rose's case, I had to add one more medication for her osteoporosis.

- Exercise is good even if you are not losing weight. It is way better than taking medications. However, start slowly.

B. **Brainstorm** the options you have.
- Afford to get a personal trainer
- Join a gym
- Organize a sports team
- Buy exercise equipment
- Start to walk/run
- Exercise using your own body weight.

C. **Communication**
- Communicate with your doctor if you think you need a physical before exercise or take some precautions if you have certain medical conditions.
- Communicate your goal with your friends and families that they can be cheerleaders for you and also keep you accountable.
- Communicate with deep you to make sure what you really need and what you want to achieve. Keep yourself motivated.

What is my exercise target?

It is really hard to define. Generally, I recommend my patients do moderate-intensity exercise every day for at least 30 minutes. Certainly, if you can do more, it will be better. However, each exercise target should be individualized. I have patients who do manual work, and after work they are very tired. For these patients, I ask them to focus more on portion control.

.

Do I need to buy wearable technology to track my activity?

If you can afford one, it is a good idea. It has been shown to motivate people to stay on track. I have one, and I show my patients that I have been doing my exercise every day. This also motivates me. There are many different brands and prices though most are doing the same thing. You can just buy the one you can afford. Otherwise, I recommend creating an exercise journal.

Chapter 11. Misperceptions about Weight Loss

Weight loss is about dieting. Is it true that if I follow a diet then I can lose weight and keep it off?

Weight loss is like doing something else. You need to be clear why you want to lose weight. You need to have a purpose. If you just want to lose weight, I bet you will be discouraged and even if you are able to lose weight you will gain it back and more in no time.

You need to keep your reason for losing weight fresh, whatever it is, but it should be strong enough that wakes you up and drives you to do the things you are supposed to do. I want to be a good doctor and add value to my patients' lives. I want to educate my patients because I believe life is the patient's life. These days, 80% of diseases are patients' diseases (my estimation). In other words, patients have to heal themselves. Hypertension, heart disease, diabetes, hyperlipidemia, obesity, fatty liver are all one disease and it is patients' disease. It is caused by patients' poor lifestyle. Patients, you have to heal yourselves. I wake up every day 3 to 4 am. I research, reflect, and collect.

Before you start your weight loss journey, write down why and ask yourself if it is strong enough. Dieting is maximally 40% of it. I think the why should be 40% of it.

Weight loss is not easy and keeping it off is harder. It is like any aspect in your life.

Remember:

- Live easy, your life will be hard.
- Live hard your life will be easy.

If my insurance pays for gastric surgery, then weight loss will be easy. Is that true?

It is true that gastric surgery is very effective in losing weight. However, I see so many people regain their weight 5-10 years later even after surgery.

Surgery helps you reach your goal, but you still need to work on it to maintain it.

For those patients, if they continue to eat poorly they will not be able to gain weight. They have more trouble with severe mineral vitamin deficiency. Their health is not better but worse.

I need to snack or eat 6-7 times a day. Otherwise my body goes into starvation mode and I will not be able to lose weight. Is this true?

This is not true. You need to have some time of fasting, so your body has the opportunity to burn the fat in your body. If possible, I recommend people to fast at least 12 hours a day.

I also recommend patients fasting periodically just on water and leafy vegetables once or twice a week. It is very helpful especially for patients suffering from severe hypertriglyceridemia (the triglycerides are too high in the blood).

I started to walk. I should be able to lose weight.

Walking is very good and burns some calories and increases your metabolism rate. It needs no equipment. It doesn't cost money except buying a pair of good walking shoes. However, walking is very low intensity exercise. It doesn't burn a lot of calories.

For a 200 lb person, walking a dog 60 minutes only burns 95 calories.
If you eat one apple, it has 95 calories.

For a 140 lb person, walking a dog 60 minutes, only burns 60 calories.
If you eat one single grape, you need to walk 4 minutes. If you eat 10 grapes, you need to walk 40 mins.

If you eat a medium blueberry muffin, it has 426 calories. In other words, you need to walk 4 hours 26 minutes to burn the muffin.

Now you can see, if you do not control your diet, walking alone will not help you lose weight.

Are only Americans getting fatter?

You might think only Americans are fat. It is not true. We as the human race are getting fat.

I found the following information on the New Zealand Ministry of Health website:

The New Zealand Health Survey 2016/17 found that:

- Around one in three adults (aged 15 years and over) were obese (32%).
- An additional 34% of adults were overweight but not obese.
- 50% of Māori adults were obese.
- 69% of Pacific adults were obese.
- Adults living in the most deprived areas were 1.5 times as likely to be obese as adults living in the least deprived areas.
- The adult obesity rate increased from 27% in 2006/07 to 32% in 2016/17.

For more information, please google the New Zealand Health Survey.

Are Asians doing better?

Not true. The numbers look better because they use the same standard of BMI to measure Asians. They need a different standard.

If the right standard is used, Asians' obesity rate is increasing at an alarming rate.

Let us look at one obesity complication-diabetes.

In India in 2017, the Indian Council of Medical Research sponsored study suggests the widespread seriousness of diabetes across rural and urban areas with some areas showing prevalence as high as 13%. To put this into perspective, the diabetes rate in America is around 9.4%.

Let us look at China's statistics. A large, nationally representative survey in 2013 of adults in China found that the estimated overall prevalence of diabetes was about 11% and that of prediabetes was nearly 36%, according to a study published by JAMA (The Journal of the American Medical Association). In urban areas, the diabetes rate in adults is as high as 35.7%. In the 1980s, the rate of diabetes was estimated below 1%. Again, put into perspective, the American diabetes rate in 2018 is around 9.4%.

Asians are not better. They are worse. We just use the wrong measure.

Chapter 12. Mindful Living-Identify the Bad Habits and Form the Good Habits and Lifestyle

What is a habit?

A habit is something we do over and over again without actively thinking about it. Every day it is estimated that at least 45-50% of the things we do are habitual. Research after research has shown that habits have tremendous effect on our lives.

Good habits help us live healthily, and bad habits lead to obesity, diabetes, fatty liver and lower our quality of life significantly as well as cause premature death.

Is there any study about health habits and mortality?

Lester Breslow and James E. Enstrom started a study in the 1960s and followed for a decade in California. They identified the following seven "good habits": never smoking cigarettes, regular physical activity, moderate or no use of alcohol, 7–8 hours sleep/day regularly, maintaining proper weight, eating breakfast, and not eating between meals. They found that men following these seven health practices had a mortality rate of only 28% that of men following zero to three health practices. Women following seven health practices had a mortality rate 43% that of women following zero to three health practices. Both the health practices themselves and their relationship to mortality were shown to be reasonably stable over the ten-year period of follow-up.

What are the bad habits?

The bad habits are endless. The good news is that we know the good habits.

Do you know the quote "All happy families are alike; each unhappy family is unhappy in its own way." The good habits are similar, and the bad habits are endless.

Practice the good habits and you will know the bad habits.

How to identify the bad habits?

As we know, habits are the repeats we do not really think about. The best way is to use "mindful living".

Set up a day, or a week to be aware of what you have been doing. Write them down and evaluate and identify the good habits and bad habits. Then work on them one by one. The most effective way to get rid of a bad habit is to replace it with a good habit.

Can you summarize the good habits?

-Eat an appropriate amount of food-portion control of meat and carbs.
-Eat all varieties of colorful, non-starchy vegetables.
-Maintain an active lifestyle.
-Maintain good emotional control and good stress management.

How are habits formed?

Four components are identified: cue, desire/craving, habit process (thought or action) and reward. This loop has to be processed a few times (some people say over at least 21 days).

However, whether the habit can be formed or not actually depends on the following function.

The strength of the cue (F(c)), and the strength of the personal desire (F(m), the strength of the social environment F(s), the difficulty of the process F(d), and the reward F(r).

Habit=F(c)+F(m)+F(s)+F(d)+F(r)

Each of the above functions can be plus or minus. The more positive, the more likely the habit will be formed and ongoing.

If you want to break the habit, you want to make the more negative possible. If you want to form a habit, you want to make the more positive possible.

How to make the F(c) cue more negative?

The F(c) can be the function of our five traditional senses: sight, sound, touch, smell. taste. F(c) can result from other nontraditional, but easy to understand, senses like balance, acceleration, deceleration, pain, sexual stimulations, cues from internal organs, etc. F(c) can also result from time, thought.

If you want to stop a bad habit, you need to reduce the F(c) cue as much as you can.

The most sustained way to reduce the F(c) cue is to remove yourself from the environment.

The examples are:

- Your cue for you to eat fruit is to see some laying on the countertop. Remove them, put them in the refrigerator. I do not recommend snacking even on fruit.
- Your cue for dessert is the smell from the cookies. Do not bake those cookies.
- Your cue for alcohol is stress. Mindful understanding the stress and reducing it is the key.
- Your cue for junk food is going out with your friends. Do not go with those friends.
- Your cue for overeating is going to a buffet place. Do not go there.

How to make the F(c) cue more positive?

If you want to form a new good habit, you need to make the F(c) cue more positive.

If you want to start an exercise habit in the morning, you can start and maximize a cue using the above senses- like visual. Post a note to yourself where you can see it. Set up your exercise outfit/gear in front of your bed or in the bathroom; audio-you can use an alarm clock or smartphone; touch- set up a pair of exercise shoes in front of your bed; smell-you can set up a scent to release when you get up to remind you.

How to make the F(m) motivation more negative?

If you want to stop a bad habit, you want to make the F(m) motivation more negative. The motivation is closely linked to F(r) reward. You need to make the reward less attractive.

One way is to magnify the unpleasantness of the habit.

For example, if you want to quit smoking, it is recommended to have mindful smoking. In the process of smoking, you are recommended to fully appreciate the taste, the smell. People said they are disgusted.

Another way to reduce the motivation is to link the result of the habit with another unpleasant feeling. Let us use smoking as an example again. You can link the smoking habit with the disapproval from your kids or your spouse.

The most difficult and most sustainable way to reduce the F(m) motivation is to move the long-term effect to the front. For example, you want to stop the bad habit of bedtime snacking. If you can move the long-term weight gain (unpleasant image in the mirror) or joint pain to now, your motivation to eat a snack at bedtime is going to reduce. However, not so many people can do it.

How to make the F(m) motivation more positive?

If you want to form a new habit, you need to make the F(m) motivation more positive.

Most good healthy habits do not have an immediate reward.

Here are my recommendations:

- Give a thought reward to yourself when you complete your "forming" habit. Here is what I do. I don't really like exercise, but I exercise every day. After I finish my daily exercise, I give myself a "thought reward" like " I finished exercise for another day", " I can tell my patients-I am doing exercise every day; I am able to conquer my own weakness; I am able to conquer my laziness; I am able to move my long term benefit to present; I am able to proudly say I am practicing what I preach..."

- Move long term benefit to the present. Let us say you want to start a new habit of eating vegetables every meal. You can make your vegetables tastier and you will be rewarded right away. You can make the long-term benefit more current such as having better bowel movements, and you might also lose weight.

How to make the F(s) more positive?

F(s) measures the social influence. This can be the combination of your social culture, community and your friends. It is not so easy to change the social culture, but it is possible to change your friends.

If you want to start taking a dancing class, you might want to ask your friends to join you. It is much easier for you to stick to it if you have a good friend going with you.

You can make your community healthier. I recently went to China, and I saw they have taken up Square Dancing. After dinner people came out to an open space and began to dance.

Michelle tried to bring more fruit and vegetables to school and promoted the benefits of fruit and vegetables.

How to make the F(s) more negative?

If you want to break a bad habit, you need to make the F(s) more negative or at least neutral.

If you want to break the habit of going to the bar after work, you can talk to your friends beforehand that you want to stop drinking and ask them not to call you. You also can choose to cut them off.

Campaign against junk food. This is another example.

How to make the F(d) more difficult?

F(d) measures the difficulties of a habit. Usually the bad habits are easy. If you want to break a bad habit, you need to make it more difficult.

If you want to break the bad habit of eating ice cream, stop buying it. When the time triggers your desire to have ice cream, guess what, you do not have it. If you really want to have it, you have to drive to the store to buy it. You make the habit more difficult. Most times, your desire/craving is going to stop.

If you want to stop the bad habit of overeating, you can do the following to make it more difficult.

- Only prepare a limited amount of food. If you want to have more, you have to restart from scratch.
- If you go to a restaurant, ask the server to pack half of your meal first and give it to you when you leave. If you want to eat more, you have to ask your server to unpack it and this will embarrass yourself.
- Use the smallest plate at home and at a party.
- Do not go to buffet places because there is so much food and it is so easy to get more.

If you want to stop snacking after dinner, you can do the following.

- Certainly, the most efficient way is not to buy what you usually snack on. If you want to eat, you do not have it. If you really want to eat it, you have to go to the store. You make it so difficult and you just give it up.
- Another way I do is to brush my teeth right after dinner. You feel better and if you eat snacks then you have to brush your teeth again.

If you want to stop the beer drinking habit, the best way is again not to buy it.

How to make the F(d) easier?

If you want to start a good habit, you want to make it easier.

We all want to exercise every day. As a matter of fact, this is in most common new year's resolutions. Not too many people follow through. One problem is people make the habit too hard. Instead we need to make it easy.

I have a patient who was very excited and came to tell me that he joined the best gym in town. Three months later, I asked about exercise. He was embarrassed. He was not really going but was still paying. What happened? He needs 15 minutes to drive over there, and 15 minutes driving back, plus changing clothes and afterwards showering 20 minutes. If he exercises for one hour, he needs nearly two hours to accomplish this habit. He does not have this much time.

Here is what I recommend for exercise.

- Many work places have gyms. It may not be the best, but it is the most convenient. You do not waste time traveling to and from and you do not need to exert much effort to go.
- Find a gym on your way to work if your work place does not have one.
- If you do not have either, you don’t need a gym. You can buy equipment to use at home. If you want to buy one, the most useful ones are elliptical machines or stationary bikes. They are the best. Most people can use them. Treadmills are not the best. I do not recommend people running on them since there is too much impact on the knees and hips. Many people are injured.
- Exercise doesn't really need to be done in the gym, or by buying equipment. You can do it anywhere and anytime. It would be great if you can talk to a physical therapist for some ideas.
- Exercise all the big muscle groups, not just repeat one movement. In this way, you will not be getting bored but also more effective. I go to a gym to exercise in my work place every day. I do at least ten different machines so this way I am able to accomplish my exercise routine relatively easier.
- Distract yourself. When I do my exercise, I listen to a book, or watch TV. The time goes by so much faster.

Chapter 13. How to Conquer Hunger

What is hunger?

Hunger may mean different things to different people. Here we are talking about hunger which is a discomfort signaling you to seek food. It certainly can come with different intensity.

Hunger can be a successful diet barrier. Hunger is very complicated involving nerve transmitters, hormones and peptides. Some other conditions or diseases can also cause hunger. Boredom and stress can both cause hunger.

What are the possible conditions causing hunger?

- Gastrointestinal (GI) conditions such as ulcers, gastritis or gallbladder conditions including cholecystitis or stones. It is common for people who have a stomach condition to feel hunger more often than people who do not have these conditions.
- Your blood sugar is low.
- Taking some medications like steroids.
- Hyperthyroidism, 10% can have weight gain. Please read my book about hyperthyroidism.
- Some rare conditions-see Chapter 22.

What are your suggestions for combating hunger?

1. Find out if you truly are hungry especially if you have diabetes and are being treated with medications. Check your sugar. If your sugar is > 100, the chance of you having real hunger is low.

2. Not to drink ice-cold water. Ice-cold water "shocks" you stomach and makes your stomach sick and you mistake it as hunger.

3. If you have diabetes, balance your diabetic medications and your food intake. If your sugar was under reasonable control before you started to diet, most likely your medications need to be adjusted.

4. Not to eat simple carbs which can cause a condition called "reactive hypoglycemia", then you need to eat more to raise your sugar. Certainly, this does not help you lose weight.

5. Try to balance your meal better. You can replace your red meat with white meat such as chicken, turkey breast, egg white or fish.

6. Try to balance the intervals of eating. I do not recommend snacking. But if you are the person who is struggling with hunger, I recommend you take four meals a day. If you are diabetic, you need to let your doctor know if you would like this option. Your doctor would adjust your medication especially insulin accordingly

7. Use vegetables as snacks. Good options are celery (no dressing), broccoli, cauliflower. Even carrots are better than cookies. You can steam or boil to soften your vegetables. You can also add some flavor to it as long as not too much salt, or fat.

8. Next option is to drink some hot drinks such as hot tea and black coffee.

9. Vegetable soup. Basically, you can boil/steam/braise the vegetables you like and add any seasonings you like. You can also add some chicken broth to get the taste. **You can add a few pieces of meat/shrimp. For some people meat is more effective in curbing the appetite.** Portion control is the key.

10. Tomato egg drop soup. -- I found this recipe is very healthy and can help you deal with hunger. Tomato has high levels of lycopene which was reported to increase a hormone level called adiponectin which increases insulin sensitivity. It is very easy to cook. Water- amount depending how much you want to drink, raise to boil. Cut one medium sized tomato and stir in one large egg white (if you do not know how to separate the egg white from egg yolk, please search a YouTube video). Total calories from this soup is 40. This soup can last you for two hours.

11. Snack with some nuts. Most nuts (no salt or honey added) are okay, 10-12 pieces are the limit.

12. Some fruit-- half of medium sized apple, one small orange, five medium sized strawberries.

13. Drink some fiber(prebiotics). You can buy fiber supplements from store online or offline.

14. Consider appetite suppressants. Right now, we have a few medications which are approved by the FDA to suppress your appetite to help lose weight. Some medications work from brain. Others work from the gut. For more information, please refer to Chapter 23.

15. FDA approved a new hydrogel pill-Plenity, which makes you feel full but no calories. It is expected to be available in the US in 2020.

Chapter 14. Conquering Boredom

Case presentation

Joe works in a local grocery store as a shelf-stocker. He came to me requesting a testosterone shot. He is 45 years old and divorced six months ago. In his weight history, he gained 30 lbs after the divorce. He attributed his weight gain to eating all the time out of boredom especially at night. He could not stop eating while watching TV.

What is boredom?

Boredom is a common feeling or emotion of emptiness and yearning to do something more stimulating or meaningful.

Two characteristics are very important. One is the emptiness feeling, and the other is wanting to do something about it.

What are the causes of boredom?

This is actually built in our genes. We are built to make ourselves better, the people surrounding us better and our environment better. If you are not doing any of these, you will feel bored and want to make changes.

What is good about boredom?

Boredom is actually a drive for communication, person to person connection (relationship), socialization or innovation. Some artwork is also created from boredom. Think about it. If we didn't get bored, we might just be very comfortable sitting or lying in bed doing nothing.

Why does boredom lead to obesity?

Boredom makes people uncomfortable. Many of us choose the easy way out by eating. Eating is easy and something fun and satisfying. The dopamine (the happy neurotransmitter) fires right away and makes you feel better. Suddenly you are not feeling bored any more. Some people also turn to drinking. Some people even do both (drinking and eating). Some even do drugs. They are using boredom the wrong way.

How do you recommend to fight boredom?

First: boredom awareness. When aware of boredom, people realize it is not hunger. Snacking is significantly reduced.

Second: doing something is the key.

Third: For the long term, start a new hobby or a new project.

What are your recommendations for fighting short term boredom?

You can go have a run or go to a gym. This is the best.
Go outside to have a walk and enjoy your environment.
Talk to your neighbor.
Call your friend/family.
Clean your house or apartment.
Read a book. Go to the library.

If you have some talent like singing, dancing, or playing an instrument, this is a good time for you to practice and get better. If you do not know how to do any of these things, it may be the best time to start.

What are your recommendations for fighting long term boredom?

- Start to play a musical instrument. Anyone can start to learn. I know someone who started to play the piano at age of 72 and he became pretty good at it. When you play music, your brain and hands will be too busy for snacks.

- Start a new hobby. Think back to when you were younger. You might have liked to do something, but later your life became too busy. Now you can start again.
- Start a garden. You can plant some vegetables for yourself.
- Start to learn a new language. I knew a patient whose ancestry was German, but he did not know how to speak German. He was bored and frequently snacking. He was not able to control his diabetes and weight. I ran this idea by him, and he took it. He was able to speak German in a year. He took his children to visit Berlin and they were so impressed with him and really admired him. He felt very good. Now he also has native German-speaking friends, thus expanding his social circle.
- Explore your curiosity. We are all curious about how things are working. Pick up a subject that interests you and start to study it. Many adults are not good at computer science. It could be an opportune time to learn some computer science.
- Volunteering is very good. You are helping other people. This makes yourself better.
- Working. Nothing is wrong with working. If you think you can handle another part-time job, go for it. I have Steve who took my advice and found a part-time job working at Home Depot. He earned more money for Christmas gifts for grandchildren, learned new skills, met more people. He actually lost weight, since he was sitting down to eat all the time. Now he is busy and forget about snacking. I have Justin who is a retired engineer. He retired at age of 65 and I saw him for his diabetes at that time. We tried everything for his diabetes, and insulin made his sugar up and down. He was certainly gaining weight. It turned out that he was so bored at home and snacked all day long. Finally, I advised him to go back to work. He did. His company was really happy to hire him back since his skill was in demand. Now he actually was so much happier, and his sugar was stable. He was able to lose the weight he gained after retirement.

Chapter 15. How to Cope with Stress

What is stress?

Stress is part of life. Stress is your body's response to the changes of your living environment, your body, or your thoughts. It was "designed" to protect your body.

Why do you talk about stress in this book?

More and more studies show that maladapted chronic stress causes prediabetes, diabetes, obesity, fatty liver and cardiovascular disease. Maladapted chronic stress also causes an array of psychological and physical illness including but not limited to hypertension, heart attack, stroke, anxiety, depression, insomnia, antisocial violence…

In my daily care for my patients, I see what stress has done to them. Stress sends diabetes out of control, blood pressure out of control, weight gain, anxiety, insomnia, depression, among other things.

Stress could be the number one cause for obesity. Everyone eats under stress.

How does good stress become bad?

Stress originally was designed to help our body deal with "emergencies". People refer to stress responses as "fight or flight". It enables your body to get to safety and you have harmony again with your environment.

However, in modern society, we do not have lions to eat us, but we feel like we're being attacked from all over the place. We do not feel safe. At the same time, we feel that we do not have a place to "flight", nor do we feel empowered to "fight." Thus, stress becomes chronic.

Because, we feel powerless, we resort to "wrong ways" of adapting to stress to alleviate the "pain of feeling being threatened." We resort to using aggressive behavior by attacking people physically or emotionally, by withdrawing (depression), or to food, and drugs. Harmony cannot be reached between the inside and outside of your body.

Why does maladapted and/or chronic stress cause so many problems?

Stress is a combination response of the sympathetic nervous system and hormones. They all increase energy supply for your body to "fight or flight." The stress hormones are adrenaline and cortisol. Cortisol is a natural steroid.

Both the sympathetic nervous system and stress hormones increase your alertness, heart rate, and blood flow to your muscles, but constrict blood flow to your skin or other unimportant organs for "fight or flight." When the stress becomes chronic, our body needs more from the sympathetic nervous system and more steroids, but our body cannot provide more. Our body tries to adapt and use all sorts of ways to reduce the need for them.

Your brain is being over-stimulated all the time. Your brain tries to divert these chronic stimulations that lead to anxiety, depression and memory loss.

Your heart keeps being over-stimulated, and some blood vessels are being constricted. These cause heart disease and blood pressure problems.

Chronic elevation of cortisol causes your abdominal fat to accumulate because there are lots of receptors for cortisol.

Chronic elevated cortisol certainly affects your brain and stimulates your appetite. Your body wants more energy to fight "danger."

What are the stress triggers?

Any stimulants can cause your body's response to a certain degree. Your body always communicates with the changes in and outside of your body and your own thoughts to make adjustments. Stress demands your body to make changes and responses to accommodate the changes. One thing unavoidable in this world is change. They are countless. They are everywhere. They are in your daily life and can appear any time without warning.

- From your environment:
    - Your physical environment: natural disasters, war, terrorist attack, weather changes (suddenly too hot, too cold...).
    - From people: in close proximity (in family, workplace, school, church…) or far away (internet bully, cold war, being attacked on TV…).
    - Gain or loss: you build a house, or it burns down, get married, have a baby, divorce, things stolen, win or lose…
- From your physical body: pain, itching, sickness and so on.
- From your own mind:
    - Negative thoughts
    - Scary thoughts (phrase like "scared about your own shadow")
    - Afraid of losing something valuable

Can stress be good?

Yes, stress is designed to help you to meet challenges and help you survive.

Stress can increase your productivity.

Short-lived stress response is good.

How do we spot maladapted stress?

The following are symptoms and signs of maladaptive stress:

The key issue is chronic. It can mean days, weeks, months, years depending on different situations.

Chronic emotional derangements:

- Irritable, jittery, restless, feeling mad all the time
- "Kick the cat", you blame your spouse, kids, or co-workers when things are going wrong
- Withdrawn, apathy
- Feeling overwhelmed, powerless
- Anxiety, or anxious all the time

Physical derangements:

- Headache, migraine
- Palpitations, chest pain, tremor, sweating all the time
- Uncontrolled blood pressure, blood sugar
- Irritable bowel syndrome
- Restless syndrome
- Fibromyalgia (feeling pain all over your body)
- Panic attacks
- Poor memory, lack of concentration

What is the most positive way to respond to stress?

First, let us face it, everyone has stress. Stress can sometimes be a good thing. Research has shown that people under some stress improve productivity. However, stress, if not properly handled, can cause very detrimental effects in your life.

The best way is to prevent stress turning into bad.
When you meet a difficult situation, always tell yourself that it is a challenge, but I am in control. You are in control. This doesn't mean you have to "fight". You can choose "flight". Another option is to accept the situation and you then have the option to forget about it. You can always choose one of these options:

- To fight
- To flight
- To be free from the situation-accept the situation

Why can we turn stress from bad to good?

Most people will not have a lion standing in front of them. Most of the time we perceive the lion from which we cannot escape. The key here is that if you think you are under control, the stress is helping you to accomplish your challenge. If you think you are not under control, and being at the mercy of "the lion," your body is under siege and stress becomes chronic. This is bad.

Our minds are very powerful. We can change our perception by thinking or talking. The reality does not need to be changed. Your sense of control can be changed. Your body's response can be changed. Stress can be changed from bad to good.

How can we turn stress from bad to good?

Based on research I read and my experiences with my patients, and myself, I developed the following key points in preventing bad stress from happening or turning bad stress to good stress.

Step 1: identify the red flags of stress becoming bad. Read the question above about the symptoms and signs of stress going bad (How do we spot maladapted stress?) Sometimes it can be very challenging. You might truly have a physical illness. You might need a doctor to make the diagnosis. For example, I have patients with hyperthyroidism that can cause many symptoms of stress maladaptation; I also have patients with an adrenal tumor called pheochromocytoma (tumor secreting adrenaline) who can have similar symptoms and signs of chronic maladaptation of stress. There are many more diseases which can cause similar symptoms and signs. If you are not sure, please see your doctor.

This step is very important. When you know it, you can tell yourself. Ha, ha, now I am under stress. This is the way my body prepares me to meet the challenge. This is your mind taking control of the situation itself by recognizing you are under stress.

Step 2: Identify the source of your stress.
When you feel stressed, and you are overwhelmed, you need to slow down, sit back and try to identify the source of your stress.

This is the way to tell yourself that you are in control.

Step 3: Analyze it to see if there is anything you can do about it. In other words, see if there is something you have power to change about the situation or not.

Choose an option:

- Fight
- Flight
- Free- to accept your situation.

For those things where you think you can make changes, go ahead and do something instead of sitting there worrying.

For those things you do not have the power to change, just free yourself and let them go.

For those things, you cannot let go, then you just “flight.”

All options are good options and the truth is that you actually do not know which one is best.

The most important thing is to make a decision and stick to it with effort for a reasonable time.

Step 4: Preemptive preparation. For those stressors which you can predict, start to prepare early. The more prepared, the less stress will be. I cannot be prepared for everything, but there are more things that can be prepared for ahead than you think. Therefore, every time, when you feel really stressed, write down the stress. Ask yourself, next time, can I be more prepared?

Step 5: Do not assume more responsibility than you can handle. Sometimes, you have to learn to say NO. I have a patient who is a very hard worker. Every time her boss asked her to do something she always said yes. She had to work more and more and put too much pressure on herself until one day she had a nervous breakdown. Think about it. The boss certainly wants you to do more and more, so he or she can make more money. You have to stand up for yourself.

Step 6: Exercise. Exercise is a good way to release stress. Running, walking, you can do anywhere. Swimming is very good. You repeat strokes and get your mind off the stressors. Most people feel relieved.

Step 7: Do something you like or start a new hobby. Some people like playing music, singing, drawing, horseback riding, reading, hiking. Doing something else usually can get your mind off your stressor. If you like video games, go play some video games.

Step 8: Talk to your friend or your loved ones about it. Sometimes, talking about it brings relief.

Step 9: Ask for help if you can. Ask for help from your loved ones, friends or anyone if you think might help you. You never know until you try. It does not cost much to ask.

Step 10: Position yourself at the right place. Do not put yourself at too high of a position. Realize your limitations.

Step 11: Focus on other people. Go help someone else, and you will realize that there are many troubles in the world, and more unfortunate people than you are. Plus, when you help other people, other people will help you when you need it.

Step 12: If you believe in God, pray and give your worries to God. He will help you.

Chapter 16. Coping with Stress from Children and Grandchildren

Are you as an Endocrinologist equipped to give advice on this topic?

"Happy families are all alike; every unhappy family is unhappy in its own way." Author unknown.

Over the years in talking with my patients, I have heard so many stories relating "tragedies and stresses" from raising a child (children). There are so many situations which I cannot imagine. Sometimes I felt unequipped in many situations, since these social issues have many legal implications, need resources, and have particular circumstances. I felt as powerless as my patients. Many times, I wanted to omit this chapter. However, I think some of my own reflections and knowledge gained from my reading and research might be helpful to some parents.

My advice comes from the following:

- I have a girl and boy. I have had my share of stressful situations the same as other parents.
- I grew up with my children! In raising my children, I made lots of mistakes, but I learned and made changes.
- I have heard hundreds of stories from my patients.
- I try to put my feet in my patients' shoes and ask the question: what would I do?
- I read parenting books.
- I read child growth and development research and books.

What are the options to dealing with the stress from children?

The basic options for dealing with any stress situation are:

- Fight-try to embrace your stress and overcome it
- Flight-ignore it
- Free-try to change yourself and not be bothered

Many people will tell you what you can do or not do and be legal. Here I am only giving the options.

We know we want to be a good parent and fight. I agree and most parents are doing just that.

Here I want to share two cases about -" flight". I am not saying you should give up, but life is more complicated than those moral judges and laws.

Case: This story came from a grandma who is my patient. She said this happened to her close friend's granddaughter. Let's give the close friend's granddaughter a name- Emily. Emily fell in love with a boy during her junior year of high school. She got pregnant while a senior but was able to manage to graduate. She moved in with her boyfriend to an apartment. Soon after her graduation, she gave birth to a beautiful girl. They had some help from both family and government but not enough. They were stressed in dealing with the child's crying, day care and needs for themselves. One day the boyfriend took off and did not come back for two days. Emily was so mad, and the child cried continuously. She was not able to take it anymore. She boiled water and poured the boiling water onto the baby from head to toe. My patient went to take care of the baby while in the hospital. The scene was so horrible. My patient prayed every day to let God take her. She died in five days.

I was in shock hearing this tragedy.

What if Emily said, "I have too much stress in taking care my own child. Can I give her away for adoption?" I think if Emily put "flight" as an option on the table, this tragedy might not have happened.

Here I have another story.

Case. I will give a little background: China used to have a one child per family policy. Also, people thought only a son could keep the family going. There was strong conflict. One side, people wanted to have a son. Another side the one family one child policy was very strict. If you violated the law, your job would be taken away, your house would be torn down. Some parents could not accept the fact of having a girl and had lots of stress. They chose to "give away" their own girls. Many of them were adopted by Americans.

Morgan Hurd was one of them. She is the 2017 World all-around artistic gymnast champion, a member of the gold-medal winning American team at the 2018 World Championships, and a five-time World medalist. She is a three-time member of the United States women's national team (2016, 2017, 2018).

She was adopted from China when she was 11 months old. I do not know the situation of her birth parents or what went through their heads. One thing I know is that they had lots of stress and they chose to give her up and gave their daughter a chance to live and live to her fullness. Morgan also has made her adoptive parents so happy and proud.

I have a toddler at home, and he is very difficult to manage. What can I do?

Toddlers are really fun but also can be very challenging.

Case. Marilyn is my patient and I am seeing her for hypothyroidism. She has been trying to lose weight but instead she has been gaining weight. She has been juggling between her job, housework, and taking care of the toddler. She has been really stressed. It turned out that her toddler was very challenging. He always says NO, made a mess in the supermarket, and threw a tantrum. He does not want to go to bed at bedtime. Every day she feels she is fighting a battle with her toddler. She feels powerless and exhausted.

Again, let us use the technique A, B, C.
A: A represents Acknowledge

- This is normal child development.
  - Children around the age of two begin to realize that they are separate individuals from dad and mom.
  - Children begin to have strong emotions, like happy, sadness, anger, joy, fear, etc. However, they still do not know how to express them with language (we adults often do not use words very well either).
  - Children at this age still do not understand logic or consequences. They do not understand the future. This means that when they want something it means now. We adults sometimes act the same. We want it and we want it now!

- This is an opportunity to learn more about your child, a moment to experiment your way of teaching and help your child and yourself to grow. When you change your attitude toward these challenges, you will look at these challenging moments as fun. Read a parenting book and experiment with some techniques and see if they work or not.

B: B represents Brainstorm options. In any stressful situation, calm yourself and think about options. You always have options and quickly evaluate them. Learn from other parents or from a parenting book. There are numerous options and theories.

C: Communication. Toddlers understand more than we think.

Case. Marilyn was at my office. She got a call from daycare. She was apparently distressed. We formed a game plan together. She was told that her toddler bit another child in fighting for a toy. She was really mad because she was stressed with her job already. She wanted to spank him, and yell at him and put him in a closet. Luckily, she now knows better. She took a deep deep breath and composed herself before leaving the office. She had a game plan before going there mad.

- Acknowledge this is normal in child development. Her child is not the first child who bit another child in history.
- Acknowledge that her child needed to express himself.
- Acknowledge this is an opportunity for her and the child to grow. She has this opportunity to control her own emotion of anger and frustration. This is also her opportunity to teach him how to get what he wants and learn how to share.
    - Now she is thinking if his child does not master the skills of sharing, communicating, and team playing, this similar thing might happen in the teenage years. At that time, he might be more powerful, and not just bite other people. He might punch other people or stone other people for what he wants. Or even kill other people.
- After this, she is really calm and confident to go to the daycare to face the teacher, other parents, and her child.
    - To the teacher: she did not choose blaming. (Why didn't you watch more closely? What were you doing at that time? You were paid to watch my child!) Instead she is very apologetic and graceful.
    - To the other parents: She apologized on behalf of the child. She did not try to belittle or exaggerate the incident. She just apologized for what had happened and went home to work on it.
    - To the child: She did not yell at him or shame him, threaten him, spank him. She just got him to another room and asked what had happened and asked him a few questions like "Do you like

somebody to bite you?" "Is it right or wrong to bite another person?", "What should you do when you do something wrong?", "What can you do next time if you want to play with a toy someone else has?"

My son has trouble with his grades. I am worried that he might not be able to get into college. What can I do?

Again, I like to use A, B, C.
A: Acknowledge the reality:

- My son is not good at school. Some people are good at books. Some people are not. My son may be just one of them.
- Luckily, college is not the only way leading to making a living, and certainly not the only way to be happy.

B: Brainstorm the options.

- There are many options like going to trade school to become a mechanic or electrician. FYI, salaries for mechanics and electricians are higher than most college graduates.
- Starting a business. Lots of successful stories are out there.

C: Communicate with him to see what ideas and plans he has for himself.

- As parents it is very natural to worry about them, but they may already have a plan. The only thing we need to do is to ask.
- If they have no clue at all, it is okay to make suggestions.

Case. Toni is a 40-year-old single mom. She has never been to college. She has been working two jobs and trying to provide for her son. She has been stressed about her son's grades since middle school. She hired a tutor and did whatever she could do, but her son's grades were still not good. He even may not be able to graduate from high school. Her dream for college for her son just broke her heart. She has been really stressed.

She came to see me for her thyroid and weight gain. I helped her with A, B, C.

She felt so much better and realized this is not the end of the world nor the end of her son's future. There are many ways leading to success and happiness. As parents, we want our kids to be self-sufficient and happy. College is just one of many options.

Now she is not so stressed and communicates better with her son. She actually enjoys being around her son. Her son's grades actually improved, and he graduated from high school. He now went to a trade school.

My teenage girl is dating a boy which really worries me. What can I do?

I thought teenage dating and sex were not stress triggers any more to American parents until a grandma came to me stressed about her granddaughter.

Case. Mae is a 72-year-old grandma. I am seeing her for diabetes. Lately her sugar went up and she gained weight. It turned out that she had been stressed over her granddaughter. She and the parents tried to separate her from the boy. The tension at home was very high and they still failed. One night, they all went to bed and the girl sneaked out and climbed into her boyfriend's house through a window. Grandma is really stressed about her granddaughter who is very smart and has good grades in school. She was expected to be the first one to go to college in her family. Her grandma was afraid that she would get pregnant and end up as a teenage mom in poverty. No one wants to see their offspring go down such an abysmal spiral.

A: Acknowledge the reality

- Times are different in two ways: the dating and sex in high school are not rare and in some schools are very common. For Mae's granddaughter it is a bit too late to give her the idea of abstinence. Certainly you can still try.
- Sex and relationships are stressful to everyone.

B: Brainstorm the options.

- Encourage her to continue to date many boys, and as a parent try to get to know them. Try to inspire the boy to study and make their lives better, so they can have a future.
- Make sure they protect themselves from STD (sexually transmitted disease) and pregnancy if they insist on continuing sexual intimacy.
- Try not to use options like "locking her in her room"-which does not work and pulls you far away from your child and grandchild.
- Try not to humiliate your child with language or hurt her with physical force. These options might get her closer to her boyfriend since she thinks she can only get support from him.

C. Communication.

- Express your love through words and action: take her boyfriend seriously and be very nice and kind to him. When you do that, she might focus on their relationship more instead of her relationship with you. She will inspect the relationship and grow. We do not want her to divert her attention to fight with her parents.
- Be alert to spot an abusive relationship.

My adult children moved back in with grandchildren. What can I do?

Case. Betty is a 62-year-old grandma. She has four children. One of them is disabled and has never left the house. Now two of them moved back in with three grandchildren. The youngest son is 29 years old. She is really stressed and no doubt she is a stress eater. She gained 10 lbs and her sugar was really out of control.

She told me that she has been living her life from crisis to crisis. Her three sons are her biggest trouble and now three grandchildren besides. She felt like she was being taken hostage by her own three adult children.

Anyone who has these kinds of children has their heart being broken. What can you do? Get them off the street and especially now that they have grandchildren. Do you want your grandchildren to live on the street? If not, what are you going to do? Your three-bedroom 1500 square feet house is filled with people. People are sleeping in the living room. Every day you need groceries and you cook for them. My patient is exhausted, and it puts lots of stress on her health and relationship with her husband. She is totally drained physically, emotionally and financially.

Initially, I gave her advice not to play tough, to show her weakness, to cry if needed. Later, I thought it over and I realized that this would never work on this group of people. They just have not grown up yet and they do not have shame, nor a sense of right and wrong. They do not have sympathy for their elderly parents.

I read a few books and one of them impressed me by Allison Bottke, ***Setting Boundaries With Your Adult Children Six Steps to Hope and Healing for Struggling Parents.*** I really encourage you to read books like this.

I organized her basic ideas into the following A, B, C.

A. Acknowledge
- You have a problem.
- You have a problem so big that you cannot solve, and you need a higher power to solve. In her book, she refers to God.
- You need to step out of God's way. You should not stand between your child and God.

- You need to do the job you need to do and allow God to do his job.
- In trying to save your child you are enabling your child's bad behavior. You have a problem. You need to make changes. Lots of parents have a problem accepting this. They all think they raised this precious son or daughter and they are trying to help them get on their own two feet.
- You can only change yourself. You cannot change your child.
- You need to live your life. You need to get your life together instead of running your child's life. They need to live their own lives.
- Let God change the adult child's life. God has his own schedule. You may or may not see the results in your lifetime.
- Your adult child has not matured emotionally. You need to give them time to mature instead of seeking to run their life. You should not feel the pain he/she is feeling.
- You need to be ready to accept whatever the result might be. Sometimes it may mean the death of your adult child. Threatening suicide is just many adult children's technique to making their parents yield to their needs and wants. They are great manipulators using fear, guilt.
- You need to begin to see who your child really is, not who you wanted them to be. This is difficult and heart piercing.
- You need to ask for forgiveness from God for interfering in teaching your adult children.
- You need to ask for forgiveness from your adult children. Your enabling behavior played a significant role in this mess. You need to realize your fault in this mess and then it is possible that you can make amends. The author suggested parents write to adult children instead of talking to avoid argument. She thinks this is very important to recognize that poor parenting choices have stunted the growth of their child and caused them to be overly dependent on the parents and to also have some pain themselves.
- You and your spouse need to have a united front.
- You need to recognize the difficulty and to have a supporting group.
- What they do with their lives as a result of our implemented boundaries will be their choice. Parents and other enablers need to recognize that we do not have control of their choices. We can only do our part. They have free will. They can make their own choices. We need to accept that fact that they may

never become someone we want them to be-productive, joyful and living fulfilled lives.

B. Brainstorm the options and be prepared for resistance from adult children.
    - Need to set up a new rule and limit the time the adult children can move back in.
    - Need to reinforce those rules.
    - Need to have strategies and planning.
    - Need to look at your life and do what you really like to do: like travel, learn a new language, volunteer, etc. Step away from your adult child's chaos.
    - Need to set up new boundaries in all aspects of life in dealing with your adult child.
    - Write them down, because you already acknowledged the difficulty. Write them down and help reinforce yourself.
    - Need to prepare and rehearse the possible scenarios.

C. Communicate your decisions and thinking to your adult children.
    - Communicate with your spouse first to achieve a united front.
    - Communicate with grandparents, siblings, aunts, uncles or well-intentioned friends who are enabling your adult children. You all need to have a united front.
    - Communication of the boundaries needs to be firm and direct but not confrontational.
    - Written communication might be better.
    - Ask forgiveness for the part you played in this mess.
    - Express your love as always. The changes you make are made with love to help your adult child to grow. It is not punishing him or her. Both parties deserve joy, peace, happiness and a fulfilling life.
    - Express that the way you have stood there to pick up the pieces of his or her life is not loving or helping. You are hurting him or her and standing in the way for him or her to grow and have a good relationship with God, and eventually to have joy, peace, happiness and a fulfilling life.
    - Let him or her know that you pray they make the right choices and accept the consequences.
    - Let them know that you believe in their ability to grow.
    - At the end of the day, following through is as important as your initial decision.

I have two children who are both addicts. What can I do?

Lousy is a 64-year-old female who has been seeing me for diabetes for five years. Her diabetes has been from okay to bad and now her A1c (an indicator of diabetes control) is over 14% (normal < 5.6%). She also gained 50 lbs over the past five years. I said: "Lousy, you have been ruining my reputation. You cannot keep your appointments. You're not taking medications, and you don't follow my diet and exercise recommendations. What is going on?" She began to cry. It turned out that she has two adult children. One is living with her and one just moved out after a fight with her and his brother. The one who lived with her was just arrested. She has tremendous stress. She is lacking the ability to deal with these two addicts. Every day is a drama. They suck out her every penny for drugs and she does not have money for gas sometimes. This is why she cannot come for her appointments. She does not have money for medication because all the money went to her two sons' drugs. If they do not get what they want, they become violent. She called police a few times, and they went to jail. They came out of jail and became even worse than before.

This has been going on for more than a decade.

I sat back and had a very long discussion with her. I want her to use A, B, C to conquer her challenge.

A: Acknowledge.

- You have a very big problem and you need God to help you. See the above question.
- You are not responsible to support your adult children for food, medical care and certainly not drugs.
- You have been enabling them to keep their drug habits. You are partly to blame, and you are not helping. Again, enabling is not helping.
- You have difficulties implementing boundaries especially when they are violent.
- You deserve to have a better life.
- You deserve to get your diabetes under better control and regain your mental and physical health.
- You have the right to pursue your own happiness.
- You do not deserve to be trapped by two adult children.

B. Brainstorm the options. We sat and brainstormed the options for her.

- Physical and emotional separation from the lives of your adult children is urgent.
- Move to another city, or move to another state, but they might be able to find you and drive over.

- Move to another country. I recommended she move to China. I know so many Americans who are living in China and they are having wonderful lives over there. The cost of living is much lower, and you do not need new skills. You have a skill of speaking English. You can just teach conversational English.
- Move to an English-speaking country. You think you will feel more comfortable, but life will be harder.

C. Communication.

- Remember, no communication is also a form of communication. Make sure not to talk to anyone your children know about your plan. These include your own parents, siblings and close friends if your children know your friends. Certainly, you should not tell your two adult children about your plan.
- If you decide to go to a country which requires a visa, you need to apply for one. My patient decided to go to Puerto Rico where she has a friend who can help her restart her life.
- You need to go to your Social Security office to find out how you can get your monthly check if you are living in a foreign country. Sometimes you might need to see an accountant or lawyer about this matter. This is important.
- You also need to communicate with your bank if you have some savings as to how to withdraw your money in a foreign country.
- You can get a lot of help from the American embassy overseas. Keep this in mind and you do not need to work out every detail before you go. To me the most important things are how to get your Social Security check and how to access your money from America.
- Talk to your doctors. Get your health care documents together. You might also need to have at least three months of medications. It might take time to set up health care in a foreign country.
- Medicare might not pay for your healthcare out of US territories.

What are the detailed steps I can follow?

If you have a troubled adult child you are dealing with, I recommend you read Allison's book yourself. I like her six-step cure for that. She used the acronym "SANITY".

- S-STOP all forms of enabling behavior (most important is money). STOP ignoring your own needs financially, physically, emotionally.
- ASSEMBLE a united front with a supporting group.
- N-NIP excuses in the bud.
- I-IMPLEMENT rules and boundaries.

- T-TRUST your instincts. If you feel you are abused and being taken advantage of, or manipulated by your children, trust your feelings.
- Y-YIELD everything to God. You need to let it go. It is not your responsibility anymore. It is God's responsibility.

What can I do with my daughter who gave birth to my grandchildren and gave them to me one after another?

Case: Abigail is my patient who is 60 years old living with her husband. Her daughter lives with one man after another and has never been married. However, she has two children who live with my patient Abigail. Basically, they adopted their grandchildren, now 10 and 13. Now her daughter is pregnant again and apparently unable to take care of the baby. She is drinking alcohol and on drugs. My patient asked: "What am I going to do?" Her husband is working two jobs to make ends meet and physically they are not able to take care of a baby. But they cannot let the baby just risk her life with their daughter.

This is a dilemma and can be very challenging for everyone. Nowadays, the grandparents and sometimes the great grandparents pitch in to raise their grandchildren, and great grandchildren. I think this is great. However, for grandparents, and great grandparents like my patient Abigail, she and her husband have lots of resentment toward their daughter. It is not easy to raise a child physically, emotionally, mentally and financially. Abigail already drained her resources but now is going to get another child and maybe more in the future.

I truly did not have a solution for my patient Abigail.

This is what I suggested.
A: Acknowledge

- That you are in distress.
- The challenges you are facing are huge and you need God to help you.
- The need for taking care of yourself.
- The resentment you have toward your daughter.

B: Brainstorm the options

- Recruit other family members to help.
- Find a grandparent support group. Again, you are not alone. The number of grandparents who are raising their grandchildren is becoming more common.

- Consider the option of adoption. There is nothing wrong with adoption, and the child can have a better physical and emotional development in a more secure environment.

C: Communication

- Okay to communicate your frustration and distress to your grandchildren but need to be age appropriate.
- Okay to assign age appropriate house chores to your grandchildren.
- Need to let your daughter know she must use contraceptives if she is going to continue living promiscuously.
- Tell your daughter you will not keep any more of her children and will seek adoptive parents.

Chapter 17. Coping with Stress from Parents

My parents are very controlling. They are very pervasive in my life. What can I do?

Case. I am seeing Robert for hypothyroidism. Lately he has gained weight. He married a year ago. They live two blocks from his parents' house. They went to the same church where his father is a pastor. His parents wanted his wife to lead a Bible study, but she didn't want to. There is lots of tension between his parents and his wife and he was in the middle. It was so bad that they had to move to another church. Since then, his parents just cut them off. It tore his heart. He is the only son and was a "good boy" and rarely defied his parents. He wants them to be happy and wants to have a relationship with them. He also wants his son to have a good relationship with his parents. At the same time, he wants his wife to be happy, too.

Over-controlling parents can cause lots of stress in their adult children's life. First and foremost is to recognize it. Here are the characteristics:

- There is only one way of doing things. That is their way.
- They know which boyfriend or girlfriend or future husband or wife is best for you.
- They know which career is best for you.
- They want everything to be perfect. They might have OCD.
- They want to know everything you are doing. They call and/or message multiple times a day.
- They want to tell you what to do and how to do it all the time without solicitation.
- You feel they are around all the time. Even if they are not you feel they are watching you.

- They feel that they need to communicate with other people on behalf of you, since they think you might not be adequate or would make mistakes.
- They make decisions on your behalf even without consulting you.
- They are the expert of manipulation using the following techniques.
    - Guilt: they really know how to use guilt. They keep saying that they worked so hard to raise you and be so good to you and your family. You are the center of their lives. You can enumerate all the things they did for you in the past and present.
    - Belittle you: you do not know what you are doing; you do not know what you are feeling; you do not know what's best for you.
    - They are expert in using bait. They give you some gift or money and ask you to go shopping and control your idea.

Then, you can do your A, B, C.

- Acknowledge your stress from your over-controlling parents. Spot the symptoms of over-controlling parents.
- Brainstorm options.
    - Set up boundaries. This is very important.
    - Empower yourself. You need to get yourself stronger physically, mentally and financially.
        - If you are sick all the time and go to the hospital frequently, or if you need your parents to come take care of you, it is very natural to nurture over-controlling parents.
        - If you are mentally unstable and cannot handle stress very well and if you call your parents for emotional support all the time, that is your invitation for your parents to step into your life.
        - If you ask your parents for money or other support frequently, it is their right to say something about how the money is spent.
    - Set up a communication distance. If you stay with your parents, you need to move out of the house. If you go to the same church, you need to go to another church. If you live in the same city, you might need to move to another city.
- Communication
    - You need to communicate your boundaries to your parents. Sometimes you need to write down your plans.

- You can expect to meet resistance. You need to be firm and prepare what to say and what to do.
- I know you love your parents, but at the same time, do not let your parents use guilt to capture you and drag you back to "old" you. I recommend you write down possible scenarios including your response.
- When your parents offer you some gift or money, you need to say no. Sometimes it is hard, but you need to be self-sufficient.
- Get your emotional support from your friends, and other uncontrolling people.
- Do not rush to answer your parents' calls. Ask them to leave a message and listen to it and think about how to respond and then call back.

My elderly parents are sick and hospitalized frequently. I am the solo caregiver. I am exhausted. What can I do?

It is not uncommon to be stressed while taking care of sick parents. If you have a few of the following symptoms, then you have too much stress from taking care of your elderly parents.

- Feeling helpless, overwhelmed or constantly worried.
- Feeling exhausted.
- Feeling lots of anxiety, palpitations, and sweating.
- Not sleeping well.
- Gaining (due to eating unhealthy food and snacking and lack of exercise) or losing weight due to depression.
- Very irritable.
- Feeling sad/depressed.
- Having diagnosis of migraine headaches, or fibromyalgia.
- Abusing alcohol or drugs, including prescription medications.

Now, after you recognize your issues then let us do A, B, C.

A: Acknowledge that you are having too much stress by recognizing the symptoms you have. Also, you need to acknowledge the following:

- It is very challenging to be a caregiver. Sometimes you may require training.
- You need to take care of yourself. If you do not take care of yourself and you get sick, your parents might be in more jeopardy.

- You need to eat right and exercise and keep your own doctor's appointments.
- You should not use food to deal with your stress.
- It is okay to ask for help.
- You cannot do everything.

B. Brain storm the options you have.

- Reduce your responsibility. You do not have to do everything. Let some unessentials go unfinished.
- Ask for help from your friend, church members and other family members. Lots of people are ready to help but they just do not know when or how. It is better to make a list of chores with which you need help. People can sign up for specific chores like grocery shopping or preparing a meal.
- Pay for a helper.
- Pay for a meal (there are many delivered meals).
- Consider a nursing home especially if your parents have special needs. Consider home nursing care.
- Find a support group for emotional support.

C. Communication

- Communicate your difficulties and challenges to your doctor. He or she might be able to provide some solution for you.
- Communicate your parents' situation to their doctor. He or she can work with you to create a feasible solution for you.
- Communicate your challenges to your parents at the level of their mental capacity.
- Communicate your needs and challenges to your friends, and other family members realistically without complaining.

My father has Alzheimer's disease. I am the caregiver and I am stressed. What can I do?

Case. Ed is my patient for diabetes. For the past few years, he was not able to get his diabetes under control and continued to gain weight. He is taking care of his 83-year-old father with Alzheimer's disease. He is really demanding and accuses him of stealing all the time. Ed is really distressed but feels very guilty if he doesn't take care of him.

We continue to recommend our A, B, C to manage stress.

A. Acknowledge

- Suffering stress as a caregiver. Read the previous question for symptoms.
- You are dealing with someone who has Alzheimer's disease. We tend to communicate with these patients the same way we communicate with normal people. They are different. You need some training to meet the challenge.
- Alzheimer's disease is very complicated. They do not just have memory loss. At certain stages, they have executive function, judgement/problem-solving issues. They forget completely how to cook and if he or she does cook, it makes it very dangerous. The most frustration comes when the caregiver tries to tell them not to cook, but they repeatedly get into trouble by cooking. They lack the insight.
- Acknowledge that the most difficulty in taking care of an Alzheimer's patient is that their behavior changes. Our emotions are naturally affected by surrounding emotions. If we are in a surrounding with sadness, we will feel sad; if with happiness, we will feel happy. If we are wrongly accused, we will be mad. It is not uncommon for Alzheimer's disease patients particularly in the middle and late stages of the disease to have behavior changes. These can begin with relatively subtle symptoms including apathy, social disengagement, and irritability. More problematic is the emergence of behavioral disturbances, including agitation, aggression, wandering, and psychosis (hallucinations, delusions, misidentification syndromes). Caregivers are distressed when they are accused of doing something wrong. We tend to think that we have been here for you and you are not appreciative and have falsely accused us. We can get really distressed. People tend not to accept that sometimes the patient talks and does things very logically. They even think the patient might not have Alzheimer's disease.
- Acknowledge the behavior of wandering. There are numerous stories where the patient leaves for a walk in the neighborhood where he or she lived for 30 years and goes missing. Missing parents can cause significant distress for their caregiver.
- Acknowledge that you are not trained for this. It is okay to feel frustrated sometimes. You do not have to feel guilty.
- Acknowledge that you can only do so much.
- Acknowledge that you also need to take care of yourself. It is paramount for you to be healthy.

B. Brainstorm options

I use the acronym Alzheimer to help caregivers remember:

- A: ask for help. Many people, friends, other family members, volunteers are ready to help. It is okay to ask for help. I recommend that you write down specific needs and ways to help. Write down more specific instructions and precautions which will be very helpful. Also warn of possible problems and how to handle them.
- L: means legal and financial. You might need lawyers or an accountant to get your parents' financials planned.
- Z: zero in on the things you can do, prioritize.
- H: means health for yourself as well as your parents. Keep your appointments with your doctors as well as your parents'.
- E: means education. You need to become an educated caregiver. As we discussed, there are many challenges a caregiver can meet. There are solutions, but education is crucial.
- I: Identify your needs and your parents' needs;
- M: meet your own physical and mental health needs. This means that you need to take care of yourself. Eat right, exercise, manage your stress.
- E: means emotions. Be aware of your emotions and improve your emotional intelligence.
- R: means resources. You need to learn about resources and manage them. The local Alzheimer's Association is a good place to begin.

C. Communication

- Keep your communication at the level of your parents' cognition.
- Keep your negative emotions in check. Our emotions are usually affected by surroundings. The patient may have negative emotions such as apathy, depression, delusion, allusion, etc.
- Do not get into arguments with your parents. Arguments don't help reduce your stress.
- Always keep in mind that your parent is a patient and you are the caregiver.
- Communicate your needs and your parents' needs to their medical care team.
- Communicate your needs to your friends and family in writing, so they know how to help.
- Write a protocol and precautions for your helpers.

Can you tell me more about legal documents and financial?

I recommend you prepare legal and financial documents early.

I recommend you find an attorney who is specialized in estate planning.

You need your lawyer's help to sort out the following:

- A **medical** or health **care** power of attorney/**advance directive**
- Property management. Some options like a reverse mortgage will help to cover personal care.
- Possible coverage of long-term care services, including what is provided by Medicare, Medicaid, veteran benefits and other long-term care insurance.
- Find out if your parent has a will. If they do have a will make plans how to execute the will. If not, get all the beneficiaries (interested parties) together to make the responsibilities and benefits clear to everyone involved.

What are the personal financial items I need to look into?

It is not easy to collect the personal financials. Sometimes, your parents might not want to touch them. When their minds are still clear, you might be able to prepare them. At the late stage of dementia, they might not know where they store the documents and what they have or not.

- Itemized list of assets
  - bank accounts
  - retirement accounts (401 k, etc.)
  - contents of safe deposit boxes
  - vehicles
  - real estate, including current value and the names listed as owners, account holders and beneficiaries (deeds of real estate)
  - life insurance policies
  - brokerage accounts-stocks, bonds, annuities and other investments
- Collect all the documents and work together with other parties who might have an interest and a financial planner/accountant.
  - Deeds for real estate
  - Will, trust, and power of attorney
  - Recent tax returns
  - Health insurance cards and booklets (you might need to research for benefits and options)
  - Life insurance (some have cash value), - you might need to evaluate to keep or cancel.

- Long-term care insurance policies or benefits booklets
- Your parents' diagnosis and treatments (past admissions)

How to reduce stress in managing your parents' financials?

It is always stressful in managing financials, even your parents' financials. Here are my recommendations. You need to work like an accountant (if possible, you actually can hire an accountant) and keep your emotions detached.

- Keep three piles of information separately: all the assets, all the income and all the expenses.
- Keep good documentation.
- Post income in the correct account.
- Pay the bills timely
    - Exam the bill for accuracy.
    - Exam the service for its necessity.
- Be creative if your parents have limited financial resources such as using a reverse mortgage.
- Communicate with an accountant or financial advisor to ensure good financial planning.
- Discuss with all parties involved to reduce the medical bills.
- Make some difficult decisions.

Chapter 18 Coping with Stress in the Workplace

Case: Steve is a 35-year-old accountant. During tax season, he is so busy. He accepted so many cases. He has been pushed by clients and family responsibility. His wife is a nurse and they have two lovely daughters 4, and 7. He found he gained 15 lbs and felt overwhelmed, had difficulty sleeping and low productivity. His wife has trouble carrying on a conversation with him. His blood pressure was also out of control. He came to me for possible hyperthyroidism which could have symptoms of anxiety and difficulty sleeping.

How common is workplace stress?

Based on reports, most of us (over 60-80%) experience some sort of workplace stress and bring the stress home. Workplace stress also has been linked to obesity.

What are the reasons for workplace stress causing obesity?

- Stress increases cortisol which is a steroid that promotes weight gain.
- Workplace stress changes eating behavior: eating faster, eating more often, eating more snacks, eating more high carbs and high fat foods, eating larger quantities, eating mindlessly.
- Workplace stress reduces physical activity. Workplace stress makes people work overtime. As we know, stress reduces work efficiency requiring more time to accomplish the same amount of work.
- Workplace stress also is linked to drinking more alcohol.

How to turn stress from bad to good?

I recommend using the following strategies. The key is to make yourself believe that you are in control.

- Spot yourself in bad stress.

  - You might feel overwhelmed, unable to focus, forgetful, making mistakes, low productivity, increased irritability.
  - Increased anxiety, palpitations, panic attacks, that frequently lead to an ER visit.
  - Difficulty sleeping, tremors, sweaty.
  - Eating behavior changes (see above).
  - Increased headaches, irritable bowel symptoms.
  - Find yourself needing to work overtime more often.
  - Find yourself arguing with your spouse or friends more frequently.
  - Find yourself gaining weight.
- Identify possible triggers
  - From your boss
  - From your colleagues
  - From overwork/too difficult work
  - From unfair pay
  - From feeling lack of control/fear of losing your job
- Weigh your options and make a decision
  - Fight-get what you want
  - Flight- resign/leave your current job
  - Free your mind-let it be, who cares?

How to change the stress from your boss?

Here, I am not talking about harassment, bullying or other criminal acts.

- Identify the possible causes: unstable emotions, too much work, treating you unfairly...
- Assess the situation and weigh the options:
  - Fight to get what you want
  - Flight (leave the department, leave the company)
  - Free your mind- accept the situation and continue to work there. Focus on what you can get from working with him/her-like paychecks.

How to fight with your boss?

You need to be prepared. You need to be prepared to leave the department or the organization. You need to prepare your strategies.

- Write down what your point is. What do you want to achieve?

- Do not talk to your boss when you are mad. Whatever happened, calm down first.
- Find a right time. Timing is very important.
- Be firm on your position.
- Talk from your boss' point of view and add more. e.g. your boss just gave you too much work, but let others play. You can say things like: "I am glad you trust me and assign me the important work. I really appreciate that. I worry that if I am sick then that important work will not be done. I have an idea. Can I train Nancy so she can take over some work when I am sick?"
- Never accuse anyone, especially your boss (here I am not talking about harassment and discrimination). Nobody likes being accused.
- Never assume. Talk about it. I have a patient who works in a sales department. She has to do all the paperwork. Lots of coworkers do not have enough to do. She was really mad. After she talked with her boss. She learned her boss did not assign some of the jobs to other people because he was trying to not offend her by assigning her work to other people.

Can I "flight" from my boss?

If you think he or she is too much for you to deal with, it might be. You have to walk away. Just walk away. I have so many people tell me that after they changed their work boss, they feel so much better. Remember not everything can be changed. Sometimes, we just have to walk away. You might worry about money to pay your bills. Again, I want you to change your worries and stress into energy to help yourself to the next level. As long as you do your job well, you will have your job, or start your own company.

Can I live with it?

Some bosses are really difficult with whom to work. However, you can free it from your mind.

- Your boss is also human and most likely your boss has a boss too. What I mean is that all humans have emotions and he or she might also have a problem with his or her boss. Your boss may just pass along his/her emotion to you. Some bosses also bring home stress to work. Check the website or other source, something may be going on. Your boss might be worried about his or her job.

- Try your best to find those triggers. Again, your boss is human and has some likes and dislikes. Find those triggers and try your best to avoid, eg, if your boss doesn't like you using your phone, try your best not to use it at work.
- Communicate beforehand. Be clear, since your boss doesn't know everything. Often, you need to educate him or her. Sometimes, you might need more specific instructions. Some bosses just look at the results; while some bosses just look at the process. They like you to do things their way. It is okay to do the things his or her way since you are the employee.
- Put things in perspective. The paycheck is the most important. So, tell yourself, I get paid. If you are happy with your customers, you can continue to enjoy them if you continue to work.

I have lots of stress from conflicts with my colleagues. What can I do?

Again, I am not talking about harassment and discrimination.

Conflicts are everywhere. As long as there are people, there are conflicts. As soon as you realize your stress is getting bad and you conclude that the stress is from conflicts with your colleagues, you need to make some decisions.

- Fight. There is nothing wrong with fight. If you do not fight, people tend to bully you. You certainly need strategies. When you decide to fight it gives you a sense of being in control. You can turn bad stress into good.
- Flight. Well, if you think you simply cannot win, just flight. There is nothing wrong with it. Workplaces are more complicated than family, but you simply might not like the culture of one company. There are thousands of companies. There are millions of jobs. Go and explore.
- Free. Free your mind from these conflicts. People claim it is easy to say but hard to do. Well, like everything else that is easy to say and hard to do, here is what I mean. You need to free your mind from these conflicts. I do not mean passively ignore. When you have a small conflict, if not resolved, it might mushroom. Here I mean you need to do something to free yourself out of conflicts.

How do I free myself from colleague conflicts?

In medicine, we like to use "A, B, C" to remember the steps to accomplish something.

A. Accept the conflicts. It is true that different companies have different cultures. You might like one culture better than another. One culture might be more in alignment with your personality. However, as long as there are people, there will be conflicts.

You also need to accept the fact that co-workers are co-workers. They are not your friends and family. It is true you spend more time with your co-workers than your family or friends. Some co-workers are like family. However, you do not need to fantasize that happening to you. You and your co-workers work together to get things done. You are learning and growing your skills and you get paid.

This is very important. After you accept this, you then can start to look at this as an opportunity to improve your problem-solving skill. As soon as you start to look at it as a challenge and not a problem, your stress will change from bad to good.

B. Brainstorm the cause of colleague conflicts. There are many causes. Each conflict is different. Consider this as an opportunity to improve yourself. You would evaluate yourself to see anything you can improve. This is how you grow. You would consider:

- Do I impose my value system on other people?

  We all grow up in different families, different environments. We have different perspectives on life.

I have an interesting story to tell you.

A little background information: Confucianism is like a religion in China. The core teaching is that if a king practices virtue, the whole kingdom will follow it; the parents practice virtue, the children will follow.

Zeng Guofan was a general at the end of the Qing dynasty. At that time, he was leading an army fighting the Taping Rebellion. He practiced Confucianism as a religion. He did not just practice it himself but required his army and co-generals and the emperor to do the same. At the end, nobody wanted to work with him. As soon as the Rebellion group was calmed down, he was demoted and sent home.

After a few years of self-evaluation in the countryside, when the Rebellion was recouped, he was called to serve again. This time, he only required himself to practice Confucianism. He actually accepted bribes and gave bribes to get things done. These were absolutely "no no" in Confucianism. He was able to unite other generals and the army and to keep the Qing Dynasty at least half a century longer.

- Do I need to control my ego (self-importance)?

  Mason is a 46-year-old software engineer who works at a local company. He has been working there for a decade. I have been seeing him for his diabetes for a few years. He came back with high sugar and weight gain. I asked what was going on. He told me that he was under tremendous stress. His group recently hired a few young people and now suddenly he became an outsider. He was left out even for going out for lunch. He also began to worry about his job. When he is stressed, he eats more snacks and does not take care of himself. He grew more anxious and his work efficiency was reduced.

  I asked him "Do you really know that your company is planning to lay off people?" He said, "No". I said "You might just put yourself ahead too much. Let's brainstorm what really happened recently at your workplace."

  He was able to tell me that he was very upset when those youngsters (his son's age) told him that his way of doing things was not the best way. He was really offended. This could be the starting point. No one likes to be told that their ways of doing things are not good. We take pride in the things we do. However, there is always a better way. This is how the world progresses.

  I talked to him about his ego and how to control it. In the few weeks after, he was able to reduce his ego and asked the youngsters for suggestions. He was able to get more work accomplished and he was able to blend back into his workplace.

- Am I jealous of other people?

Jealousy can ruin any relationship. This is one of the most negative emotions. It is your normal response to seeing something your peers get and you do not.

Jealousy can cause you to say and do negative things to your peers. People definitely feel your negativity very quickly.

Emily and Amy were hired by a company as human resource managers at the same time. They were best friends in college. In a few years, Emily was promoted, and Amy was not. Amy tended to say bad things about Emily. She deliberately made mistakes and blamed Emily. In the end, they became worst enemies instead of best friends.

Jealousy can be very sneaky. You need to be extremely vigilant.

- Am I bad-mouthing other people?

People are prone to gossip. Especially if you are jealous, you want to put other people down and raise yourself up. No one likes to have people gossip behind their back, but the person gossiping could be you.

My number one rule is never saying anything negative about other people. You know he or she will know in no time. If I do, I also show other people that I am not confident in myself. Instead, I am trying to raise myself by putting other people down.

- Am I not sharing credit?

It is human nature to want to grab all the credit, but who wants to work with you? They want you to work by yourself. Sometimes they even sabotage your work. Nowadays, we are only part of a project. We lost the direct connection from doing the work to results. People tend to feel more important than they really are and exaggerate their own part in the work. If you are a manager, it is important to acknowledge other people's hard work. People are more concerned about their own position than the whole project.

- Am I an accuser?

Remember you do not like to be accused. No one likes it. If you like to accuse other people of bad things, certainly they won't like you which creates workplace tension.

- Am I not able to control my emotions?

  We are humans and we have emotions. Like at any work place, we will have things to be mad about, angry, jealous, depressed, and so on. There are negative and positive emotions and generally speaking, anger is not a good emotion to show.

  When you show your anger, the communication channel is shut down between you and your colleagues. Tension and stress are increased.

- Am I giving other people reasonable doubt?

  Things can be very complicated. What you see and hear may not be the complete picture.

  Be slow to make judgement or draw conclusions. It is very important in dealing with workplace relationships to not label people.

  I want to tell you another old Chinese story about Confucius.

  We know Confucius was the most famous thinker/philosopher in ancient China. Even today his teaching is in Chinese culture.

  He had 12 disciples. They traveled from county to county, even country to country to spread their ideas. One day, everyone was so hungry and tired. Finally, they were able to get a small amount of rice. One of the disciples named Yanhu cooked rice for everyone.

  Confucius walked by and saw Yanhu eating rice sneakily. Confucius did not accuse him of eating rice and instead asked how the taste was. Yanhu was really embarrassed and told Confucius the fact that when he was cooking the rice some ashes contaminated the rice. Because rice was so precious, he did not want to waste any. He was eating rice with ashes.

  This story shows us that sometimes when you see something is happening, it may not be what you think it is.

C. Communication.
We all know the importance of communication. We all need to improve our communication skills.

Here I want to emphasize the following:

- Don't rush to conclusions. Be patient to hear what is really being said. The skill of repeating back is very useful. When you repeat back, people hear what they are saying and tend to calm down and explain it better to you.
- Try not to argue. Most times, arguing will not work. Arguments increase people's emotions and they become very defensive. The better way to change other people's ideas is to be open-minded. This means you are ready to accept other people's ideas. Instead of trying to say more, you need to listen more and say something like, "tell me more", or ask questions.
- Accept other person's feelings. Most of the time, different people have different ideas because their "benefit" is being breached. However, you should not say that. You need to just acknowledge that this is important, and listen.
- Apologize if you can. We are humans. We all make mistakes. Apologizing does not mean your motivation is wrong or bad. You can say, "I am so sorry that what I did (what I said) hurt you. I should have paid more attention to what words I used when I said that. I should pay attention to what you might perceive about what I did."

Do not try to explain first. You need to apologize first. Your colleague will calm down much quicker if you apologize. When you explain and give justification, people usually will become more aggressive and defensive.

I will share my own recent experience. Our clinic is going through a lot of turmoil. One day I went to my colleague's office to see him. I was waiting at his nurse's office. He stayed in the exam room for a long time. I began to talk to his nurse. Then during the conversation I said he was talking too much. I waited a few minutes more and then I left since I had my patients to see. Then at night, I got an angry call from him. "Are you my friend? Did you say I was talking too much?" He was really mad. First thing, I did not try to explain. I just listened and tried to understand what was really going on. Often, people are mad because there is something else going on and they only heard part of what you said. I first apologized that what I said made him really mad. Then I asked if anything else was going on. Then he told me that he also heard that somebody said, “He was losing his mind.” I am not going into too much detail here. My point is that people are interpreting what you do or say based on their own context. After I listened to what he said, I apologized to him again because I was not careful when I made that comment. Then I explained to him that I intended to say that he was a good doctor and spent time with his patients.

What is ego?

Ego is part of Freud’s three-part theory of personality.

Ego is sense of yourself. It is unconscious. When it is being attacked, you automatically become defensive. However, when you become defensive, then the other party is also becoming defensive. There will be two armadillos in the room.

I have been trying to form a new habit to combat this automatic reaction. Every time, when I feel I am attacked, instead of trying to explain or attack back, I say; “tell me more…”, or I repeat what he or she said. When your attacker hears this, usually they calm down because they sense you are listening.

I also try to learn and grow myself. I pay attention to other people’s responses and learn other people's skills.

How do I know if I am jealous of my co-worker?

Besides the symptoms and signs of stress listed previously, you might also have the following symptoms:

- Very critical of your co-worker
- Talk bad behind his or her back; spreading rumors
- You use the tone of satire very often.
- Feel very insecure.
- You withdraw from co-worker social functions.

How can I reduce jealousy of other co-workers?

We all know jealousy can ruin relationships and make you act irrationally in a contact with your co-worker. Here is what you can do:

First, as we stated. acknowledging it is very important. Be vigilant and spot what you have been going through.

Second, you need to realize that the basis for jealousy is coming from a big assumption and premise that we are equal and that we should be treated equally. For example, when Donald Trump goes somewhere, he has secret service and when you go out you have to ride a bus unprotected. You never have a sense of jealousy over this. Why? Because you do not think of yourself equal to the president. You are jealous of your co-worker because you think you are equal. You might have the assumption of equality in your education, your age, your work ethics, your achievements, and so on. However, in reality, there could be more. Your co-worker might have some social connection the company needs. Your co-worker might have worked harder and smarter and you did not see it. Your co-worker might have better negotiation skills. Your coworker might have better communication skills, but you did not appreciate them because you are busy being jealous. Or simply there is only one position and only one of you can have it, and your co-worker has the position and not you.

Third, focus on improving your skills and continue to do well in your job. Be receptive and ready for other opportunities or seek new opportunities. By the way, you never know if the position you are seeking actually is good or bad for you anyway.

Here is an example. I have a story of Elaine Lan Chao, current Secretary of Transportation. I heard her story from one of her talks.

She was born in Taiwan and immigrated to the US while in primary school. She studied banking and transportation at Dartmouth and Harvard. Before she got an intern position in the White House, she worked for Bank of America.

She has very significant experience in banking and transportation. In 1986, Chao became Deputy Administrator of the Maritime Administration in the U.S. Department of Transportation. From 1988 to 1989, she served as Chairwoman of the Federal Maritime Commission.

She worked hard in George W. Bush's campaign. When he was forming his cabinet, everyone predicted that she would be nominated for Secretary of Transportation and she wanted the job. This is her expertise. However, she was not nominated for anything. She did not become jealous and mad. She left the White House gracefully and wished them well. She left to work for Bank of America again. Later, she was nominated as Secretary of Labor because the first nominee Linda Chavez withdrew. She became the Secretary of Labor for eight years from 2001 to 2009. She did not say the reason why she got the job. However, we can predict that if she thought that she was the best person for Secretary of Transportation, became jealous and talked badly, president Bush would not have considered any position for her.

You know that now she is the Secretary of Transportation for the Trump administration.

My point is that if you keep learning and improving yourself, a new opportunity might come to you that might be better, or you can go out and find another opportunity. Jealousy is toxic and not useful.

What can I do if my co-worker is jealous of me?

This can be hard to deal with since you can control yourself, but you cannot control other people's feelings. However, there are still a lot of things you could do:

- Do not assume. When you feel your co-workers act differently, try your best to be cool and think what you have been doing or saying that is wrong. Self-reflection is very important. It may be true that you believe too much of self-importance. It may be true that you only care about your own position. It may be true that you forget to acknowledge other people's efforts on the team.
- Communicate but do not confront. Choose a right moment. You had best inquire into what is going on and ask for advice to improve yourself. Try not to confront your co-worker because it does not work. It can only increase the tension and make your co-worker very defensive.
- Help your co-worker to grow. One of the reasons for jealousy is people's insecurity. If you help them grow and improve, their feeling of security will increase.
- Give your co-worker credit when deserved. We all tend to exaggerate what we contribute and forget other people. When you are ready to acknowledge your co-workers' contributions, they will calm down and work better.

- Forgive. This is also very important. Try your best to understand where your co-worker comes from. Insecurity is the main reason for jealousy. If your co-worker bad mouthed you, try to let it go and move forward. Try to think what you can do to improve yourself.

Chapter 19. Dealing with Financial Stress

What is your general recommendation for money management?

Someone said: "Money isn't everything, but it's right up there with oxygen." I totally agree with that. I think you do, too.

I am not a financial advisor. I never make money by investing. The following ways to deal with financial stress just come from my own life wisdom. This advice is not for those people who think they need a investment/financial advisor or want to become a millionaire.

- Find a job that pays more. I always hear that it is so hard to find a job. One is very lucky to have a job. The truth is that as long as you want to work, you can always earn more. Here are several key issues.
  - Do your job well. Don't just do your job, do it well. When you become an expert or the best who can do the job in your company, if you ask for a raise, you will get it more often than not.
  - Keep learning. It is very important to learn new skills. When you have new skills that is your capital. When my son was a high school student, the first job he had was in an ice cream store. He earned $8.00 per hour. He likes computers and he learned to repair computers himself. Then he found a job in a computer repair shop. There he earned $12.00 per hour. He then found himself a sales associate job in an Apple Store. He was paid $15.00 per hour and got a few shares of Apple stock in his account before he went to college. He worked very hard. His sales doubled the second top sales associate in that particular store.
  - Keep looking. One day, I met someone who really surprised me. He moved here from another state. He did not know anyone in town, but he wanted to earn more money. He likes

baseball. After the game, he went to the office and asked how he could get a job as an usher in the stadium. Instead he got a job selling alcohol at a concession stand. One season, he earned $100,000 dollars just in tips!

- Find a side job. You might think you do not have any skills. There are plenty of jobs which do not need skills such as at a grocery store at the check-out line--help with bagging. If you can work 8 hours a weekend, you might be able to earn $80 extra per week. $80 can do a lot of things.

- Look for help. You might need to talk to a social worker to find any government or community program out there for which you qualify. There are all sorts of programs in America to help people get back on their own feet. Some of them are group specific, such as veterans. Most are not group specific. Again, ask a social worker.
    - **For medication, please ask staff in your doctor's office. Many drug makers have programs to help people who cannot pay**.
- Do not assume more financial responsibility than you need to.

It is not uncommon for parents struggling to pay for their son or daughter's college tuition. You know you do not have to assume this responsibility. They need to assume their own responsibility.

- Reduce expenses. Look at your daily life and you will find that you can cut down a lot and still be happy. Do you know about "low carbon living" which means "green"-consume less and help our planet.
    - Ask the following questions:
        - Do I need such a big house? You know you pay extra for mortgage, taxes, utility bills (more to heat or cool), more time to clean.
        - Do I need to have a big car? Small cars use less gasoline. These days, gasoline is very expensive too. Used small cars also have smaller tax and insurance bills.
        - Do I need to have cable? You might need more time to work instead of watching TV any way.
        - Do I need an internet connection at home? Look into the options of going to the library or some store for internet connections. If you can eliminate this, it can save you at least $40 a month.

    - Do I need a smartphone? Smartphones are expensive, and a data plan is expensive. Most of the time, we really do not need one.
    - Keep thinking, you might have other ways to eliminate some expenses.
    - Here is what I did to cut down my expenses. We eliminated the cable which cost us $60/month; we stopped our land line which cost us $20/month; we stopped our internet which cost us $90/month; we also stopped Amazon prime which cost us $120/year. I saved $190/month.

- Stop bad habits.
  - If you are smoking, it is a good time to stop. A pack of cigarettes is $6 or more. If you smoke, a pack a day. In a year, you can save $2190. This is a lot of money.
  - If you get a cup of coffee from Starbucks every day, stop. At $6 dollars a day, you can save another $2190. Most are not healthy anyway.
  - If you drink alcohol, stop. Here is another $2190 in a year.
  - If you buy lottery tickets, stop. I know it is really tantalizing to see people winning. However, I am sure for you it is a losing business. If you spent $10 a week on the lottery, you will save $520.
  - If you drink soda, stop. Soda is sugar and carbonated water. This is bad for your health. Drinking water can save you at least $10 a week, and $520 a year.
  - Stop looking for sales. Stop browsing sale websites. You know that everything is on sale! You will be tempted to buy lots of things you do not need simply because they are on sale.

My medications are so expensive. I have to choose between medications and food. What can I do?

Case. Billie came with her husband Bill. Bill is my patient. I see him for diabetes and high cholesterol. He is on Toujeo (a kind of long-acting insulin) which threw him into the "donut-hole" very quickly. He also had a stent which was put in by his cardiologist last month. He was started on Brilinta. Now he is paying $1300 for medication every month. Both of them only earn less than $2000 a month. They are tapping savings to help but their savings are depleting very rapidly. Both of them are really stressed.

We use A, B, C to tackle this problem.

A: Acknowledge

- That you have too much stress from your financial burdens.
- The stress might cause more harm than the benefits the medications can provide.
- There is always a way to resolve your challenge.

B. Brainstorm the options.

- Make more money. Start a side job if you can.
- Seek help from family and friends.
- Cut other costs, such as downsizing your house which can save a lot of money (reduce your taxes, utilities and maintenance cost), get rid of unnecessary stuff.
- Change medications. There are always different generic, less expensive medications which have similar effects and might reduce side effects.
- Eat better, and exercise which might have better effects than your medications, or even eliminate the need for medications.
- Read my recently updated diabetes book. You can find lots of resources (websites) to reduce your medication cost.

C. Communications

- Talk to your family about your difficulties. You never know some of them might be able to help. Some family members may have a charity budget. You might become their charity.
- Talk to your children and grandchildren even if they do not have money for you. They might be able to help do some chores and cut down your cost. If they help you mow the lawn, you will save some money. If they come to drive you to a doctor's visit, you save money. Most important, they will not expect you to give them gifts during the holidays. Managing expectation is very important. If you do not say, they do not know. Sometimes, unnecessary tension might come from unrealistic expectations.
- Talk to your doctor about your difficulties. For the short term, some doctors might have samples or coupons to help you. Most of the time, you can use a generic version. Sometimes, the new version might be slightly better or sound better but in reality, it is questionable. The huge price you pay may not be worth it.

Case. Go back to the above case of Bill. We discussed more about lifestyle changes and also motivated him to do more on that. He was able to quit snacks and reduce his portions. The most important thing is that he was able to quit smoking. For his diabetes, after a few months, he lost over 30 lbs, and his sugar was much better and meanwhile I provided some samples. Then I switched to Novolin N which was $24 dollars every 1000 units. He also talked to his cardiologist and he was switched from Brilinta to clopidogrel (generic for Plavix). Quitting smoking saved him $1500 a year. His risk for recurrent heart attack or stroke reduced by at least 50%. There is no other "drug" which can have so drastic effect. He also breathed better. Now he does not have a money problem and feels better.

- Talk to yourself to see if you can do better on modifying your lifestyle.

  Case. I have Jim who is a 66-year-old male who came to me for diabetes. His fasting sugar was 230, and his A1c was 10.2%. His BMI was 42 and he also showed evidence of fatty liver. He retired early. He was on at least ten different medications. I changed his insulin regimen and provided some samples. When he came back in a few weeks, he felt better with better sugar control, but he was sad and disappointed to tell me that his insurance did not pay for the medications I prescribed, and it would cost him $2000 more. He already used all the money he can use on his medications.

  I told him the truth that if he could do what I said, he would not need any insulin and many other medications. He actually was able to do it. Over 1.5 years he was able to lose 80 pounds and he is using minimal amounts of insulin. I provided many samples and he was able to reduce his other medication. He also felt so much better.

- Again, ask doctor, staff, fellow patients about help resources from foundations, pharmaceutical companies, etc. If you happen to have diabetes, read my recently updated diabetes book. I have listed many resources to help people like you.

Holidays are approaching. I always stress about finances during the holidays. What can I do?

Case. Sophia is a great grandma. She is 72 years old. She has seven grandchildren and three great grandchildren. They are so lovely, and they are her life. I have seen her for her diabetes and blood pressure. She spends a lot of money on healthy eating and medications. She is living on a fixed income and really does not have too much money to spare on holiday gifts. Christmas is coming and she felt that she had to give them nice gifts to show her love. She really was stressed. Her sugar and weight are up.

Taking care of diabetes is very expensive. Copays, deductibles, donut holes, you name it. As a doctor, I feel the pain every day for my patients. Many patients have to cut down on their medicine to put food on the table.

Here are my suggestions to help you reduce your holiday financial stress. Let us use A, B, C again.

A: Acknowledge

- Acknowledge that your excess stress is from your worries about financials.
- Acknowledge that overspending during the holidays is from your excessive expectations for yourself.
- Acknowledge that during the holidays, you do not owe anyone a gift.
- Acknowledge that gifts are not the only way to express your love.
- Acknowledge that your children, grandchildren, or great grandchildren love you not because you give them gifts.
- Acknowledge that purchased love is always cheap and will go away if no gifts are given.

B. Brainstorm the options.

- Always let your doctor know if you cannot pay for a certain medication. Most of the time, your doctor can find another alternative which may be more affordable. Your doctor might have some coupons and samples to give you some relief.
- Let your family and friends know that you are in financial trouble. They might have a charity budget. They might be able to help.
- Reduce your holiday giving list. Honestly, most gifts are useless anyway. You do not need to give everybody a gift. Even if they are expecting it, you do not have to give it. You can say you are sorry that you are not able to buy them a gift this year. Tell them you are stressed financially, and that you need the money to buy medicine for diabetes.
- Buy gifts while they are on sale. If there is someone you feel you have to give a gift to, you do not have to wait to the last minute. You can buy a gift after Christmas for next year's Christmas.
- If you have talent, you can make a gift yourself. It will be much more valuable and more meaningful. Believe it or not, your gift receiver will

appreciate it more since you put more thought into it, and you get a chance to show off your talent.

- Start a new tradition like a family gift swap. It is fun and you do not have to buy everybody a gift. It cuts down a lot of waste and saves a lot of money.
- Set boundaries to give gifts to your children, grandchildren and great grandchildren only and younger than 18 years old.

Case. Avery is an 82-year-old female. I actually also see her husband, Ben, for diabetes. Christmas is approaching. They have lots of stress from her granddaughter. They had only one son who died in an automobile accident. Now his daughter is 16 years old. Every Christmas she requests a very expensive gift which is over their budget. This year, she already requested an iPhone x which costs more than $1000. Avery and Ben are really stressed about this. Last year, they tried not to meet her request. After going back and forth, they had to give in and gave her an iPhone 8. She is very manipulative and takes pity on herself that if her father was still alive, he would give her a new iPhone and now she doesn't have a father, and nobody loves her. Avery and Ben felt guilty and gave in. Now this year, she requested another more expensive iPhone. My advice is to set up boundaries in facing people who are manipulating your emotions, love and loss. It is never a good idea to buy your love. As we discussed in a previous chapter, you are actually not helping her learn about money.

- Find a side job if you still can work. Working is good for your weight loss and diabetes. Certainly, being over stressed from working is not good either.

C. Communication

- The most important thing is to communicate with yourself and manage your own expectations. You do not owe anybody gifts and you do not need to be stressed over unnecessary things.
- Communicate with your doctors and they might be able to help your end of year medications.
- Communicate with your potential gift recipients to let them know that you are in financial stress and not to expect gifts.
- Communicate with the people who usually give you a gift. Since most gifts are useless, just let them know money would be more useful.

Chapter 20. Coping with Stress from Your Spouse

Case: Elaine, a 45-year-old female, came in with a ten-pound weight gain and uncontrolled diabetes.

She had lots of stress lately. Her husband had cheated on her and they were on the verge of a divorce. On one side, she felt betrayed and did not want to live with him anymore; On the other side, she still loved him, and they also have two teenage girls in high school. She also has not worked for the past ten years. She is afraid of going back to work.

Case: Bill, a 50-year-old male, came in with sugar in the 500s.
He saw me two years ago. We were able to help him lose weight and brought his A1c down to 6%. I asked what was going on and why I have not seen him for two years.

It turned out that he was in a messy divorce and his company is trying to push him to retire. He is reluctant for his wife to go and reluctant to leave his job.

What he was doing was not working and in no time, he probably would be dragged into the hospital. He had visited the ER two times already for high sugar and high blood pressure.

I told him that we have to embrace changes because changes are inevitable. We actually do not know what is better for us in the future.

I told him a story of a Chinese farmer and his horses that I read in my primary school.

In the old days, a farmer had a horse that ran away. His neighbor came over and told him, "I am so sorry to hear your horse has run away. This is really unfortunate."
The farmer said, "Maybe."

The next day the horse came back bringing ten wild horses with him, and in the evening his neighbor came back and said, "Oh, you are so lucky and now you have eleven horses!"
The farmer again said, "Maybe."
The wild horses were wild. The following day his son tried to ride one of the horses. He fell off the horse and broke his leg. The neighbor came over again and said, "That is really unfortunate."
The farmer responded, "Maybe."
The next day the officers came around to force people to enlist in the army, and his son was saved because he had a broken leg. Again, his neighbor came and said, "Isn't that lucky!"
Again, he said, "Maybe."

The lesson of this story is that we really do not know what is good for us or not. Things happen, let them happen. I have so many high school classmates, who were not able to get into college, and now quite a few became millionaires!

Our relationship is in crisis. What can I do?

Remember what we do for stress. Remember those three options:

- Fight: do whatever it takes to repair your relationship
- Flight: leave your relationship
- Free: don't let it bother you

I asked Elaine that deep question "do you still want to live with your husband?" She said no but still worried about the future of their two girls and getting a job.

Making the decision is crucial. No one really knows what is going on with your relationship. The key is to make a decision. The stress is coming from non-decision.

Elaine divorced her husband and you know what? Eight months later she is dating again and working in a local supercenter as a cashier, but she is happier. She is planning to go back to school to be an accountant.

In America, there is a 50% divorce rate. You are not alone. Things do not work out. So be it. Move on.

I want to fight for my marriage. What can I do?

First you need to make sure that your partner has the same thinking, or you are able to convince your partner.

Then, whatever happened between you and your spouse, there is nothing wrong with working together to repair your marriage.

Our former president Bill Clinton and his wife Hillary Clinton worked out their differences and up to today they are still married. No one knows what is really going on between you and your partner. Only you can make the decision.

Devote yourself to improve your skills in dealing with disappointments from your spouse and lack of insecurity from yourself. Devote yourself to improve your skill of love.

When should I get marriage counseling?

In reality, every couple needs to go to a marriage counselor. When things are going well, who cares, until things are going badly. Again, 50% of American couples end in divorce and some are very messy.

The best time to get counseling is when things are going well. Prevention is so much better. When in a crisis, in reality no one listens to anyone. I heard one couple went to marriage counseling after a big fight. The counselor asked them to write down the negative parts of their partner. They could not stop writing. This might help but in most cases it does not really help.

A good analogy is that if you want to repair the roof it is better to choose a sunny day. It is also true for marriage counseling. It is better to have it when both of you are calm. When you are calm, you are more receptive to other people's ideas and opinions.

What can I do to reduce my stress in marriage?

As we solve all other relationships, this is easy to say but hard to do.
A, B, C

A: Acknowledge

- The difficulties of marriage. Marriage is made in heaven but must work on earth. You need to work on it.
- That marriage is not the fantasy of romance. Lots of marriage discord comes from the fantasy of romance. Romantic love does not need to work, instead just sit at the beach under the sun! You do not need to make dinner and as a matter of fact, you do not need to eat. The reality is that after sex and the unexpected product coming is a crying baby, you will have an extra life between you and your lover. You have to be responsible for his or her life.

Here I want to relate a most horrible story that I heard from my patient. Linda came to me distressed from uncontrolled diabetes and gaining weight. She had lots of stress. A horrible thing happened to her family. Amelia, her cousin's granddaughter, was 20 years old and she just got pregnant from a man with whom she fell in love at first sight in an open market. The man left her before she delivered. She fell in love with her high school sweetheart later. They moved together and in no time, a beautiful little girl was born. It sounds like a good story with a happy ending. This happy ending started a tragedy.

Tragedy happened. After the baby was born, both lovers were distressed. They found there was no music but baby crying; there was no beach, but endless house chores; there were no soulmates, but only fighting. The boyfriend did not expect this, and Amelia did not expect this. One day, the baby would not stop crying. Amelia was really frustrated and asking where the romance was she dreamed of. She thought it was all because the baby took it away. She shook the baby violently and the baby lapsed into a coma. The baby died in a few days. Amelia fled. Both her family and police did not know where she was.

- Marriage is not the fantasy of two souls melting together. The reality is that two totally different people live together. Even two people who were born in the same family and grow up in the same family are different people. You might have siblings. Think about them. Are they the same as you? They are not. Now two people born to different parents with different education and in different environments, you should expect these two people to be different. You should expect that people are different like the five fingers on your hand. They are different shapes and different sizes and have different functions but work together to get things done. Some people might argue that that is why you need dating to find your soulmate. The reality is that life is not easy. You will meet difficulties and challenges every day and we can guarantee that you and your partner have different views on things as well as different ways of dealing with things.

Sophia and Jake are soulmates. They were also high school sweethearts. They were married for five years and they have a three-year-old lovely girl. Now they are fighting over the little girl's education every day. Sophia thinks early music education is very important. Jake believes that it is very important to let her play and enjoy every day.

I like this quote (Author unknown).

"You come to love not by finding the perfect person, but by seeing an imperfect person perfectly."

Another wise quote:

"What counts in making a happy marriage is not so much how compatible you are, but how you deal with incompatibility."

And yet another from friend Ralph D. Winter-the founder of the U.S. Center for World Mission:

"Most people in our society marry the person they love, but the Bible says love the person you marry."

- That your lover is not your mind reader. People tend to fantasize that their lover is able to read their mind. He or she knows what I am thinking and what I want. The reality is that we all have different minds. Couples are couples but with different minds.

- That your lover is not totally a giver. He or she loves you, so he or she should put your benefit before his or hers. The reality is that your partner also thinks like this.

- That we will not enjoy sex as always. A study reported that 90% of couples have sexual discord. Men and women have different physiology. Their needs and wants are different. Plus, your environment, work, education, your culture and beliefs make things more complicated.

- That emotion is contagious. Each partner should bring home more positive emotions and less negative emotions. Be aware of now the negative emotions from outside of your marriage affect your marriage.

B. means balance. This balance is not a simple compromise. Are you satisfied with yourself in every way? I wish that I could be physically stronger and tougher. You need to balance your work and family. You need to balance your partner and kids. You need to balance your own original family and your partner's original family. There are many things to balance. Balance does not mean everything is perfect.

Charlotte came to my clinic for weight gain. She also had low thyroid (hypothyroidism). She was married to Ben ten years ago. Now they have two girls and one boy together. They have their hands full. Every day she is very busy taking care of her family, but her husband is still not happy. She said he still accuses her of not doing this and that. She has lots of stress and worries about her marriage.

After a few minutes talking, I learned that Charlotte had put all her energy on her three children, so her husband felt neglected. They even rarely have sex. We talked about how to balance kids and husband. I suggested that sometimes she also needs to treat her husband like a fourth child. I know it is too much for her, but that is what she needs to do to save the marriage. I wish I could also talk to her husband. Unfortunately, I am not a marriage counselor.

Here is another patient's story. Noah came for low T and weight gain. He is a young lawyer. He has lots of work every day and sometimes he has to travel out of the states. He has two kids and a lovely wife. Lately he and his wife are fighting all the time. He thinks that he works so hard to provide everything for the family. He is expecting a peaceful and restful place, but in no time, it turns into a war zone. He thinks that his wife is not appreciating but complaining about everything. After more inquiry, I learned that he works too much and needs to pay more attention to his wife and the kids. Later, I did treat his low T, and became his "marriage counselor".

I want to tell another interesting story to show the importance of balancing your work and your partner. In the past five years, I have had two such cases.

One day I was consulted in the hospital for Ava who was admitted for low sugar. She is a 45-year-old housewife. She was found by her husband at home to be confused. The ambulance brought her to the ER where she was found to have sugar of 28 (normal around 100). After workup, I found out that she injected herself with insulin to induce low sugar deliberately. It turned out that her father had diabetes and she stole some Lantus (a kind of long-acting insulin). Her husband works for a gas company and works all the time. She felt neglected and she had been sending signals to her husband, but he did not respond, so she risked her life to get more attention.

C. certainly means communication. You can learn a lot from the internet for free and from your marriage counselor by paying. Here is what I have learned from my own marriage and my patients.

- Use words. Do not fantasize thinking your partner can read your mind. This doesn't mean both of you can't create a "secret language" to communicate. I read in a novel that when the husband wore blue pajamas it meant he wanted to have sex; and when the wife put on red pajamas it meant she wanted to have sex.
- Use the right words. Language is everything. God created the world by words. You can create your happy marriage or destroy your marriage by words. This can never be overemphasized.
    - More praise, less criticism.
    - More statements, less blame.
    - More suggestions, less demands.
    - More "we or I", less "you".
    - More future oriented. This gives you more hope instead of regret or blaming.
- Use words at the right moments. Many people fantasize that because he or she is my soulmate they should let me say whatever and whenever I want to say. This can create a lot of problems for your marriage.

How do I know if I am jealous of my partner?

It is not uncommon for one partner to be jealous of the other. Too much jealousy can cause tremendous stress. If you have the following symptoms or signs, you need to pay attention and seek professional help.

- Feeling unloved.
- Feeling disregarded.
- Feeling your partner is suspicious.
- Feeling that you have to defend yourself more and more.
- Feeling more critical of your partner.
- Feeling insecure that your partner might leave you at any time or suspecting that he or she already decided to leave your relationship.
- Feeling that you are more depressed.

- Experiencing more anxiety, tremors, sweating, and sometimes insomnia.

What can I do if I am jealous of my partner?

Jealousy is actually not really bad. A little bit of jealousy actually helps hold your marriage together and helps both of you to grow. It makes you appreciate each other and even enjoy sex more.

Everyone's situation is different. One thing is for sure. If you are asking this question, then you have too much of it. You are in a stressful situation.

- A: Acknowledge your own feelings. By accepting them you calm yourself and can face them more rationally instead of just being defensive.
- B: Brainstorm. Think about your options.
    - You can always leave your relationship. Sometimes it might take this drastic move to calm yourself.
    - Talk to your partner. However, you need to talk to your partner as you would about a "disease" and seek a solution together. Never blame your partner by starting a sentence like "you" or "because you did this, or you did that."
    - Talk to your parents or another trusted person. We are proud and do not want to talk to other people, however sometimes talking to other people can solve our problem. We can always use other people's wisdom.
    - Read a good marriage relationship book.
    - Consult a marriage counselor. Nothing is wrong with that, since marriage actually is difficult. Lots of famous people used marriage counselors like the Clintons and Obamas.
    - Try to improve yourself. Jealousy is not good. You need to build admiration between your partner and you. It is never a good idea to let one partner grow and one partner to sacrifice.
        - Learn something new- new language, new skill.
        - Perfect your skill in art or music and get involved with some interest groups. When you are busy with your own interests, you will pay less attention to your partner.
        - Go to new places. You will meet more people and be more stimulated. Information is the key. When you own the information, you own the future. You will have the power.

- C: Communication.
  - Discuss it as a disease. I repeat-you and your spouse need to sit down to talk about your condition as a disease. Discuss your symptoms and signs.
  - Discuss in a way of seeking help and not accusing your partner.
  - Focus more on each other's feelings. Again, do not accuse each other.
  - Sometimes you may even need to see an endocrinologist to make sure you truly do not have an endocrine disease, or a psychiatrist to make sure you do not have a psychiatric problem.

What can I do if my partner is jealous of me?

Case: Mason came to follow up with his thyroid condition and I found that he had gained a lot of weight. I asked what was going on. He said lately he has had lots of stress from his wife. His wife Sofia works in the same company but in a different department. He was promoted to division chief and this was really what he dreamed for. However now his home is in turmoil. His wife became very suspicious of him and one day even came to his department to pick a fight with his female colleague and made a big scene. She accused his female colleague of seducing him.

Sometimes, things can be very messy and difficult to deal with. If you still want to continue your marriage, here is my A, B, C.

A. Acknowledge your partner and your feelings of distress. Look at your partner's behavior as a disease. However, do not say they are sick.

B. Brainstorm your options, like
   - Change your work environment.
   - Have a vacation to cool down.
   - Go to marriage counseling.
   - Talk to a mutual friend.
   - Do more things together to build more bonding.
   - Do more things to make your partner feel more secure.

C. Communication.
   - Both of you need to sit down and talk about it and admit that your marriage is hurting you.
   - Reflect about anything you perhaps did to make your spouse suspicious.
   - Make changes in the things you can change.

- Do not discuss the frustration in each other's life. The more you talk about it the more frustration you will have. It will turn into a blame game.
- Offer more help in family and professional life. If you have not been sharing household chores, you need to discuss how you can help. Doing chores together can get you together. In this case, the wife, Sofia, is also working but she also has all the household chore responsibilities. Every day she felt overwhelmed. I suggested the husband start to offer help with the household chores.
- Discuss options of doing more things together, like taking a vacation, or exercising to reduce the stress.
- Discuss some rules both of you can live with.
- Tell your partner before you go out where you are going, who you will be with and what you will be doing.
- Discuss the option of seeking professional help. In our case, Sofia and Mason went too far in their separate ways. They needed professional help.

I am impotent. What should I do?

Although 30-50% of males have episodes of impotence at certain times of their lives, you still need to see your primary care physician. However, do not let your primary care physician treat you with testosterone.

As an endocrinologist, I see a lot of patients suffering from impotence. Erection requires neural, circulation and hormonal systems intact and working together.

First, I make sure they do not have cardiovascular disease. Diabetes can cause neuropathy and vascular disease. Some people even have prediabetes and suffer from impotence.

Second, I want them to change their lifestyle: like sedentary lifestyle, smoking cigarettes, marijuana, alcohol, or drugs;

Third, I make sure they are not on medications which can cause impotence. This is actually very difficult. Many common medications can cause erectile dysfunction:

- Depression medications

- Blood pressure medications like beta blocker, clonidine, spironolactone, methyldopa, thiazide diuretics, et al.
- Ketoconazole
- Cimetidine
- Many antipsychotic medications.

Fourth, I make sure they do not have any endocrine diseases.

Case. I have a 40-year-old male patient. He came to see me due to "low T". It turned out that he had a large pituitary tumor. The sadness about this case is that his wife divorced him because of his lack of libido and erectile dysfunction. Fortunately, he married early and had two healthy sons 18 and 20 years old. Erectile dysfunction is just a symptom. We need to find out the cause if possible before treatment. Again, I emphasize here please do not let your primary care physician treat you with testosterone.

Why does my wife have no interest in sex at all (I am only talking about heterosexual)?

Couple sex discord can cause significant stress. It affects men more than women. Here I am only talking about heterosexual couples. I do not have homosexual patients requesting treatment. Every week I have couples or a female herself requesting to check their hormones or request for hormone treatment for low libido. Apparently low libido causes a lot of stress in their lives.

Libido actually is very complicated in a female. Some of the factors are listed below.

- The definition of sex is different for men and women.
- Neurologic/emotional status
- Physical conditions
- Hormonal status
- Social customs
- Childhood memories

How is the definition of sex different for men and women?

Man: sex is more like the act of intercourse.
Woman: sex is more like the act of kissing, cuddling, touching, even no intercourse. To some women, intercourse is not a necessary part of sex.

The low sex desire is determined by the patient herself. If she doesn't think she has low sex desire, she does not have the problem. In one study, it is as high as 43%.

What can a male partner do to help restore a female's sex desire?

Sex is not compatible with stress. Low sex desire can cause significant stress in both males and females. It is a vicious cycle. Both partners should look at it as a "disease".

Here are my recommendations:

- See a doctor. You can start with your primary care physician and have a health screening to see if she has a general physical condition. Any physical illness can cause low sex desire.
- Help reduce her stress. Most partners do the opposite. He tends to increase her stress by complaining, blaming, or expressing anger in other areas. Slow down and help her to identify where the stress is coming from and read my previous sections about how to deal with the stress.
- Help her with household chores to give her some free time for herself. Presently, women are still responsible for 60-90% of the household chores even when they are working out of the house.

  Case: A young couple came to have her hormones checked because the wife had low sex desire. I usually go through my above list to gain a big picture to see what we can do to help them. It turned out that physically she was healthy. They have two lovely children 1 and 3 years old. She has missed menstrual periods and was alarmed. She is a middle school teacher and has lots of stress at school. When she came home, she had to tend to two children and cook. She is also stressed at home. Every day she is exhausted. I told them that she did have a hormone problem, but the cause was stress. She simply needs some help to free herself. I asked the man to help with the household chores to free his wife, so she has time to think about sex. They did not come back for more hormone tests. I assume the husband did a better job.

- Visit her ob/gyn to see if she has gynecological conditions. Lots of gynecological conditions can cause low sex drive. She needs a yearly checkup.

Case: Susan came to me to check her hormones because of low sex drive. Her menstrual periods are essentially normal. It turned out that she doesn't want to have sex because every time she has abdominal discomfort and nausea. She became avert to having intercourse. I ordered a vaginal ultrasound. It turned out that she had a 20-lb ovarian tumor. Fortunately, it was benign. She had surgery and never came back again. I assume she is good now.

- See an endocrinologist. Hormones certainly affect female sexuality. Hormones are not just sex hormones. Literally all hormones affect the female sex drive one way or the other. Certainly, most hormone disturbances cause low libido. We all know sex hormones affect the sex drive. Other hormones like thyroid also affect sex drive.

  Case. A 35-year-old female came to me for fatigue and weight gain. She did not have menses since age of 33. One thing she is really averted to is her husband's penis which causes piercing pain. Therefore, she tried anything not to have sex which caused lots of marital and family stress. It turned out that she actually has premature ovarian failure. I prescribed birth control pills and vaginal cream. She came back for follow up. She began to enjoy intimacy again and her family has so much more peace. She literally said I saved her life as well as her family's. I emphasized that she needed to see her Ob/Gyn once a year.

- Learn a little female physiology. This is a weight loss book. This is not a sex book. However, here I list a few key points which might help you in your sex life.
  - Males have constant sex desires, day after day.
  - A female's sex desire fluctuates related to her menstrual cycle.
  - A male definition of sex is intercourse. Females have a broader definition including cuddling, stroking and clitoral stimulation.

Why does my husband not have a sex drive at all?

The male sex drive is also very complicated. It is affected by neural-hormonal and environmental interaction.

The following are common causes I have encountered:

- Fatigue (work too much or work too little)

- Stress (from all aspects of life)
- Physical conditions, not just low T (low testosterone).
- Medications (lots of medications can cause low sex drive and performance).
- Environmental factors.
- Avoidance- might have impotence and he just wants to avoid sex.

Case. I have a 44-year-old male who was referred for a possible pituitary tumor problem since one of the pituitary hormones called prolactin was elevated. His wife also complained about his sex drive. It turned out that he was on risperidone for his bipolar. Risperidone can cause prolactin to increase and thus reduce the sex hormone. He doesn't have a pituitary tumor. He was not able to stop risperidone. I started him on low dose testosterone. His sex drive was restored.

What can I do since my husband's sex drive is very strong and I do not have interest at all?

This common situation causes a lot of stress between couples. I have many male patients coming because of low libido, but more women complaining of low libido. We discussed in a previous question how to increase a woman's libido from the man's point of view. In this question, we deal with what a woman can do to deal with the problem.

A. Acknowledge this can be a big problem.
   - Your sex drive is low.
   - The sex energy of your husband has not been able to release, and it can convert to anxiety, anger, and mood changes and can also cause your anxiety, anger, and mood changes. Ultimately it will damage your relationship. It is estimated that over 75% of married couples have sex drive disparity and most of them choose to divorce. This is stressful.

B. Brainstorm the options.
   - Talk to your doctor like ob/gyn to see if you have any condition causing you to have low libido. The following conditions are ones I usually pay attention to if my patient complains of low libido.

     Conditions your doctor needs to pay attention to:

- **Sexual organ and sexual problems.** I have patients complaining of low libido because they have sex pain. Who wants to have sex if it is painful? These are the common conditions for sex pain (dyspareunia): vaginal atrophy, bacterial or yeast infection, endometriosis, ovarian tumor. Sometimes, I have to refer to an ob/gyn.
- **Other medical diseases besides sex organ conditions.** Many nonsexual diseases can affect sex drive: any condition causing general pain like arthritis, fibromyalgia, any serious chronic condition like cancer, diabetes, high blood pressure, coronary artery disease, morbid obesity, uncontrolled thyroid conditions, and neurological diseases. Some common conditions causing fatigue also need to be taken into consideration like iron deficiency, or B12 deficiency.

  Case. I had a colleague who was married just three or four years. I found that he became very uneasy sometimes and irritable. He even got into arguments with his colleagues. One day, I asked him to come to my office and pressed him to see what was going on in his life. After more than 30 minutes of beating the bushes, he finally told me that his wife did not have any sex drive at all, and he could not take it anymore. I offered to check his wife's hormones. She finally came to me. She was only 32 years old. She seemed much older. Her face lacked glowing with green and gray tones. She also had lots of other symptoms of hair loss, dry skin and very significant fatigue. It turned out she had low thyroid and very heavy menstrual periods (menorrhagia). I treated her thyroid and gave her iron infusion. My colleague was a happy man again because his wife came back to life.

- **Medications.** Certain prescription drugs, especially antidepressants called selective serotonin reuptake inhibitors, are known to lower the sex drive. Some antipsychotic medications can also cause low libido. Some pain medications like narcotics are also associated with low libido. Some blood pressure medications are also indicated.
- **Street drugs**. Marijuana can cause low libido.

- **Alcohol**. Too much alcohol certainly can cause the problem.
- Smoking.
- **Sex Hormone changes**
  Changes in your hormone levels may alter your desire for sex. This can occur from:

  - **All sorts of hormone-based birth control.**
  - **Perimenopause/Menopause.** Estrogen is trending down or is too low. Some patients have severe vaginal dryness and atrophy. This can cause significant pain.
  - **Pregnancy and breastfeeding.** Hormone changes during pregnancy, just after delivery and during breastfeeding, can reduce sex drive.
  - Too much prolactin. Prolactin is a hormone promoting lactation. It can be caused by medications, a pituitary tumor and many other reasons.
  - Too low level of androgen. Woman's libido is also controlled by androgen.

- **Psychological causes**

  Sometimes you need help from a psychiatrist, psychologist, or sex therapist. This can be very complicated.

  - Depression and treatment of depression
  - Anxiety and treatment of anxiety
  - Stress
  - Low self-esteem
  - History of sexual abuse
  - Previous negative sexual experiences

- Broaden your husband's concept of sex.

Help your husband broaden the concept of sex. A man has a much narrower vision of sex. You can try light touch, masturbation for him.

You can try oral sex. You might broaden his view by trying some sex toys. Again, you might need to talk to your sex therapist.

- Just go along with your husband and do it and fake it.

Sex is very important to a man. A man wants to show his partner masculinity. A man doesn't just want to release his sex energy. He wants to make his partner happy.

- Help your husband to divert his sex energy to something great- art, a new passion, science discovery, etc. This is called sublimation. Sometimes, it can be very successful

C. Communication.

- Sex is something hard to discuss even between the couple, but you need to put it on the table and talk about it.
- Talk about and acknowledge each other's frustration (not just your own).
- Evaluate each of the above options to see if anything is acceptable. You might have other options.
- Do not let this stress from sex evolve into other stress and disguise other stress. Face it directly.

What are your general recommendations to reduce couple stress?

In modern marriage, you need to change a few concepts.

- Wrong: Your partner should not criticize you. In reality, since your partner and you formed a "benefit corporation", you are invested in each other. Partners care more about each other and thus you tend to criticize each other more.
- Wrong: Marriage is a security and we can rest after we are married. In the era of the internet, you are being evaluated in comparison to potential competitors every day. Make an effort to grow together building the trust only both of you can have in each other. Modern marriage becomes harder and harder because we see so many alternatives/competitors.

Case. I saw Richard for his diabetes. However, he did not come back for two years. His sugar was really out of control ranging from 200-500s, and he gained weight (40 lbs) compared to two years ago.

I asked what was going on in his life. He told me that he was having a messy divorce. It turned out that they were high school sweethearts. They married after finishing college. 15 years later, his wife now became a vice-president of a local bank. He was still a clerk in local government. This might have caused his marriage to fail. Growing together is not just both having the same level of position. Both of you need to grow together in all aspects of life:

- *Work*: your career and finances.
- *Health*: your physical health. Try to eat right and exercise every day.
- *Learning*: your personal development.
- *Social*: your relationships with others; your interpersonal skills;
- *Spiritual*: your relationship with God. Need to keep up with your partner. Do not go too fast or too slow. Check in with each other often.

- Wrong: Marriage is just compromise. Most people think that as long as you compromise, you will be okay. In reality, compromise is not enough. If you or your partner compromise, you know that one of you will have frustration and resentment. People tend to take turns and if not, it is very natural that people begin to fight.

Case. Tim and Gloria were married for ten years and recently they were fighting every day. The trigger is about going to whose parents' home for Thanksgiving. Both Gloria and her mom are my patients for low thyroid (hypothyroidism). Gloria's mom has had more conditions like severe COPD. For the past five years, they always have gone to Gloria's parents' house for Thanksgiving dinner. Although Tim went along each year, he had lots of resentment. He always thought next time would be his turn. Gloria always has reasons for going to her parents' house, like her Mom's poor health. Going where for Thanksgiving is "trivial" but it created lots of tension between them because Tim has to compromise all the time. You might say so take turns. It will work if everything else works perfectly. In reality, Gloria was really close to her parents and she felt that Tim was not considerate that he won't even sacrifice a Thanksgiving for her. What kind of a husband is he? Everything has to strike equal in the middle.

The following is the conversation between Tim and Gloria if there is just compromise.

Gloria: "Can we go to my parents' house for Thanksgiving?"
Tim: "Why do we go to your parents' house again this year? We have been doing that for the last five years. Why can't we go to my parents' house this year?" He said it with lots of resentment.
Gloria:" You are so inconsiderate. It is just a Thanksgiving. My Mom does not have good health and acts really depressed if I do not go.". She began to show her unhappiness, "Marriage is about compromise."
Tim: "Why am I the person who has to compromise all the time?"
Gloria: "I compromise all the time! I did…, I did…"

They are raising tension and erupted into full-blown fighting.

You need skill to "compromise". You need to say "yes" then "and" to include yourself to make the compromise into a deal negotiation.

Case: Tim actually came to Gloria's appointment. They realized that compromise is not enough. I suggested that they can bring their parents to the other parents' house for Thanksgiving and actually they did for the next few years. Both families actually became closer in relationship. If you not only have the skill to compromise but to incorporate your needs into "and", your relationship will be happier. The conversation between Tim and Gloria will become the following:

Gloria: "Can we go to my parent's house for Thanksgiving."
Tim: "Yes, I am glad to go to your parents' house for Thanksgiving. I always love the stuffing your Dad prepared. And can we bring along my parents to your parents' house, too. They have felt very lonely lately."
Gloria: "I think this is a great idea! Let me talk to my parents." She talked to her parents on the phone.
Gloria: "They are happy to have your parents over for Thanksgiving and they can enjoy grandchildren together and share some stories together."
Tim:" Thanks so much for your parents' invitation to my parents. I think they will have a good time together."

Again, both partners need to have incorporated their needs into it and enjoy together not just compromise. This needs creative thinking and practice. Next time, when you have to compromise, be creative so that you do not feel you have compromised or are waiting for your partner to compromise.

What is your recommendation when I perceive that my spouse fail me?

For so many reasons, your spouse will fail you one time after another. If you are married, you know what I am talking about. You just want to pick up a fight. Some marriage counselors tell you that it is okay to have a fight and you might emerge stronger from fighting. I do not agree. For most people, we do not have the skill or artful way to fight and end in both parties being hurt. If repeated fighting, then lots of scars can be formed between you and your spouse and the marriage quality will determinate. So, my recommendation is trying your best not to fight. The following are more reasons not to fight:

- I heard cases died of heart attack when fighting with spouse.
- I heard cases of being "murdered" or suicide during or after a couple fighting.
- Fighting rarely can resolve the differences. What is fighting? It is attacking each other. Only thing you can be sure from a fight is that you are being hurt even more.
- I know so many times, after a couple's fighting, I ask them what you are fighting for. They even do not know the reason or it is so trivial they might laugh at if they hear that happen to somebody else. One thing is for sure. They are hurt more after a fighting.
- Read the Chinese farmer's story, you really do not know the future is because sometime the future is way too complicated for us.

  Case. I have a friend. He was married at that time to his wife when he was a policeman. The wife was really content since the policeman has good salary and pension. Well, my friend wanted to do more. He got to know somebody in the stationary business. He wanted to change his career course. The wife was really mad, and they fought all the time until the marriage was not repairable. They divorced. We do not know the future will be better or worse. In my friend's case, he succeeded and become a millionaire. My point is that what you believe in today may not be true tomorrow. You might not need to fight if wait to tomorrow.

What can I do not to engage in fighting?

At the starting point of a fight, there is always an initial attacker and one being attacked. Later on, with the "fighting" going on, this can be obscured. Both are becoming attacker and being attacked. That is why both end up being hurt.

Here is what you can do if fighting becomes immanent. Believe me, it is not easy and requires a lot of effort.

- Do and say things opposite to what your instinct wants you to do, and do it and say it as genuinely and calmly as possible. The key point is not to let your anger overshadow your message. When you are trying to do the opposite of your instinct, you need an emotion to match with it. Most likely you will not use anger. Let me give you an example.

  Case. Winston and Katrina are a couple. Katrina is a high school teacher and Winston works in an oil company and is making good money. Every day Winston comes home and sits down in front of the TV and enjoys a few beers. One day, Katrina needs help to prepare the dinner so she can send their young child to a friend's birthday party. She asked Winston's help. However, Winston was not able to get away from the football game playing on TV. He was not standing up and their child was yelling to go. Katrina was so angry and just could not take it anymore. She wanted to turn off the TV, kicked the beer and yelled at him. That was what she did. They got into a big fight. The TV was damaged as well as some furniture. The child missed the birthday party. They actually divorced a few years later. Divorce may not be a bad thing for them. Here my point is that they started with love but were not able to keep it. Here I am trying to share with you the technique to slow down your marriage deterioration.

  In this case, Katrina had all the right to attack. However, the end result was not good. Again, her intuition told her to attack Winston. If she did the opposite of her intuition, things would have been totally different.

  Here is the scene opposite of her instinct.

  Katrina put her anger away. Walk to Winston very calmly. Wrap her hands around Winston's neck and kiss him.

"Honey," says to his ear softly (opposite of yell and loud), "Everyday, the sound of the game on TV really bring peace me (opposite of annoy). I feel good (opposite of mad) when I hear it because I know you are at home and safe which gives me comfort. However, I will be happier at this moment if you can turn off the TV and help me prepare dinner." The outcome might be different. Certainly, Winston's behavior needs to be changed, but that is another point.

Winston can use the same strategy opposite to his intuition. When he was yelled at and accused, intuition/instinct wants him to fight back and that was what he did. That was the reason the small thing like cooking the dinner turned into a "warfare".

Here could be the scene if Winston can respond opposite to his intuition.

"Honey, I am sorry that I was too involved and did not hear what you said." He could just go to prepare the dinner and his wife could bring the child to birthday party. The TV, other furniture and his marriage can be saved.

So remember, when in a high state of emotion, always choose the opposite of your instinct.

- If you can't do the opposite of your instinct, remove yourself from the heated situation if possible. In the above case, neither of them can escape. As Winston, he can keep quiet and not say anything and do what his wife wants him to do. This is the way for him to escape.

- For really hot button issues, it is better to write to each other instead of talking face to face. If something requires face to face talking, it is better to have your points written down.

- Now our country is becoming more politically divided. If you have different views from your spouse and you cannot listen to different points, it is better not to talk about it.

Why is it a good idea to remove yourself from a heated situation?

In a heated situation, your emotion of anger is high. You are in the attacking mode. You need to realize that your emotions are controlled by chemicals in your body. They are epinephrine, norepinephrine and cortisol. If you continue to stay in the situation, you will continue to be in the attacking mode. You must actually take time to go back to your calm status since your body requires time to metabolize those hormones.

For the same reason, it is a little easier for the person being first attacked not to engage a fight. This is because the other person is already in the attack mode. The chemicals are already released in their body. It takes time to metabolize them. It is harder to calm the first attacker unless they really know what is going on and are strong enough to remove themselves from the heated situation.

A marriage counselor said: "In a household, you can only allow one crazy monkey at a time." I agree with this.

So if you like craziness in your household, be the first to be crazy. The second is not allowed.

Chapter 21. Medications Leading to Weight Gain and Alternatives

Case Presentation

Lilly is a 45-year-old female who was recently referred to me for "adrenal fatigue". Every day she is so tired and is really tired of being tired for so many years. She felt that no one was helping her. She has been seen by literally every endocrinologist in town. She also saw a "hormone doctor" in town and in Arizona. She brought over 100 pages of medical records and lab reports. All the hormones in her blood, urine, and saliva have been checked.

I reviewed her chart. She has over 10 diagnoses including but not limited to depression, anxiety, fibromyalgia, arthralgia, hypertension, hyperlipidemia, low libido, high estrogen, low progesterone and so on. She is taking over 25 medications and supplements. She weighs 353 lbs with a BMI of 49. Certainly, her case is very complicated, and I cannot copy the whole chart here. Basically, everything was started five years ago when she was 40 years old. The first diagnosis she received was fibromyalgia, and since then she has been on a downward spiral. She was started on gabapentin, which was not very effective, but she is still taking it. Then she was started on amitriptyline which she feels is somewhat helpful. Then later, the doctor added paroxetine for depression. Paroxetine was not very effective for her. She also began to see a psychiatrist for depression. She was started on quetiapine. Then the doctor added zolpidem for sleep. A few years later, she was diagnosed with hypertension and hyperlipidemia. She was started on medication for those. The "hormone doctor" started her on compounded estrogen, progesterone, and testosterone. She is also taking some supplements for which I have no ideas. Over the years, she gained a whopping 200 lbs. She told me that she had a two-story house. She has not been upstairs for two and a half years.

Comments:

Does she have "adrenal fatigue"? Absolutely not. This is not even a diagnosis. She is taking over 25 medications and is 200 lbs overweight. Can someone in this situation not feel depressed or exhausted?

It might take many years to unwind her situation. You look at people's medications. What is going on? This is a combination of the responsibility of patient, insurance company and doctor.

For patients, we all want quick results and an easy way out. "I want it and I want it now." We all have stress, and some anxiety. We are not working through our mental powers, meditation, exercise, talking to supporters (family and friends) but have resorted to medications. Every day I have people coming to me requesting anxiety medications and pain medications.

Insurance companies only value the procedures. If a doctor does not do a procedure, prescribe a medication or do a test, the insurance company says you did not do anything. How can you charge us? Here we are even not talking about defensive medicine. So, doctors are compelled to do something.

Doctors tend to prescribe a medication so the patient can be happy and also sound like they are doing something so they can be paid. I am not a national health care leader. Policy changes are beyond my pay scale. However, this is one of the reasons I wrote this book to help people. In this book, I focus on stress management not by using medications. I have strategies for relieving stress from your job, your boss, your colleagues. I have strategies for stress from your family, your parents and your children, I have strategies for relieving stress from coping with your financial difficulties...I am glad that you are reading this book and hopefully it will help you in some way.

What are the common antipsychotic medications causing weight gain?

The commonly used antipsychotic medications which can cause significant weight gain are the following:

- thioridazine
- olanzapine
- risperidone
- clozapine
- quetiapine
- lithium

These medications sometimes also are used to treat severe depression.

For thioridazine (first generation of antipsychotic medications), it is estimated to have weight gain of half a pound a week.

For the second-generation antipsychotic medications, the weight gain is relatively less with risperidone than the rest.

What can I do if my doctor prescribed any of the above antipsychotic medications?

You can try to do the following:

- Psychotherapy, cognitive therapy. You might need to see a psychotherapist or psychologist.
- Choose the medication that will not cause weight gain or result in minimal weight gain.
- Pay attention to your weight and start to eat right and exercise.
- Ask your doctor if you can concurrently use weight loss medications like topiramate or Saxenda.
- Ask your doctor about betahistine which was shown to mitigate the antipsychotic medication induced weight gain. Betahistine is an analogue of histamine. It is also used to treat vertigo, tinnitus and hearing loss associated with Ménière's disease.
- Ask your doctor about ranitidine which was also reported to mitigate the antipsychotic medication induced weight gain.

What are the common antidepressants causing weight gain?

Antidepressants are being used so frequently. One in six Americans are taking some sort of antidepressants. Most antidepressants can cause weight gain.

The following common antidepressants can cause significant weight gain:

- tricyclic antidepressants (in particular, amitriptyline, clomipramine, doxepin, and imipramine).
- SSRIs like paroxetine (Brisdelle; Paxil; Paxil CR;Pexeva)

What can I do if I am prescribed an antidepressant?

You can try to do the following:

- Psychotherapy, cognitive therapy. You might need to see a psychotherapist or psychologist.
- Choose the medication that will not cause less weight gain or result in minimal weight gain.

    - Bupropion is actually used to lose weight. You can ask your doctor if you can try this. The brand names are Aplenzin, Forfivo XL, Wellbutrin SR, Wellbutrin XL.
    - Fluoxetine is also a good choice. It is generic and short-term use was found to be associated with weight loss. The long-term use was not associated with significant weight gain. The brand name is Prozac; Saragem is a brand name for Prozac which is taken weekly.
    - Sertraline was reported not to increase significant weight gain in a long-term clinical trial. The brand name is Zoloft.

- Pay attention to your weight and start to eat right and exercise.
- Ask your doctor if he or she can concurrently use weight loss medications like topiramate or Saxenda.

What are the common anti-seizure medications that cause weight gain?

The antiepileptic drugs valproate (valproic acid) and carbamazepine, which are also commonly used in the management of bipolar disorder, are associated with weight gain. Gabapentin may also cause weight gain. Gabapentin is also commonly used for neuropathy, and fibromyalgia.

What can I do if I am started on an anti-seizure medication causing weight gain?

You can try to do the following:

- Talk to your prescribing physician to see if there are any alternatives for your condition.
- For diabetic neuropathy, gabapentin is my last resort. I would try vitamins and other physical therapy first.
- If Topiramate or zonisamide can be used instead, both of them have weight loss effect.
- Pay attention to your weight and start to eat right and exercise.
- Ask your doctor if you can concurrently use weight loss medication like Saxenda.

What diabetes medications can cause weight gain?

Diabetes medication is the major category of medication that causes weight gain. Ironically, insurance companies only are willing to pay for these medications:

- All insulins.
- All sulfonylureas-glyburide, glipizide, glimepiride, et al.
- All thiazolidinediones, such as pioglitazone and rosiglitazone.
- And their combinations with metformin or DPP-4 inhibitors.

What should I do if I am prescribed one of the medications for diabetes that causes weight gain?

- Try not to eat snacks while you are on insulin. Many doctors will ask you to eat snacks to prevent low sugar, but this is wrong. Eating more snacks will increase the chance of having low sugar, because when you check your sugar, it will always be high. If your sugar is always high, your doctor will increase your insulin dose because your sugar is not controlled, and you will gain more weight. For more information, please read my diabetes and insulin book(search my name in Amazon.com).
- Try to use the lowest dose possible (for type 2 diabetes). Type 1 diabetes is more complicated. You need to talk to your doctor specifically about this issue.
- Focus on lifestyle changes. Never rely on insulin to eat more.
- I recommend that you do some sort of exercise before each meal, which will increase your insulin sensitivity, and your need for insulin will decrease.
- Cut down fat intake. Fat decreases your insulin sensitivity and then your dose will need to be increased.
- Cut down on carbs. Carbs increase your insulin need.
- Ask your doctor if you qualify to use insulin in combination with some newer diabetes medications which can help you lose weight. There are the medications: GLP-1 agonists like Byetta, Bydureon, Trulicity, Ozempic, Adlyxin, and Victoza; or SGLT2 antagonists like Farxiga, Invokana, Jardiance and Steglatro, as well as their combinations.
- Ask your doctor to review your medication list to see if you can get off medications that cause weight gain.
- I do not prescribe sulfonylureas.
- I do not prescribe thiazolidinediones like pioglitazone, but now some diabetic specialists/endocrinologists are starting to prescribe them again. They believe that a small dose is safe to use.

What can I do if I am prescribed steroids?

Steroids are widely used for all sorts of conditions. If you are started on steroids, you should do the following.

- Ask your doctor for the lowest dose possible.
- Eat right-low carb and low meat. Eat a lot of vegetables, and do not snack.
- If possible, intermittent fasting can be tried. Talk to your doctor if it is safe for you to do that.
- Start exercising.
- If you have diabetes, and your sugar is elevated, you might need to increase your insulin dose, but cutting down your portions is very helpful. If possible, use SGLT2 antagonist like Farxiga, Jardiance, Invokana, or Steglatro.
- If possible, use some weight loss medications like acarbose, Alli, Saxenda.

What can I do if I am started on hormone birth control (oral, implant, or vaginal)?

Birth control has liberated modern women, but also brings some unwanted effects like weight gain, mood changes, and lower sex drive.

I recommend you do the following:

- Be sure to ask your prescribing physician about weight gain and other side effects.
- If just for contraception, a physical barrier method like a condom may be better for your health.
- If you choose oral contraceptive pills, ask your doctor if you are qualified for low dose hormone pills.
- Levonorgestrel-releasing intrauterine contraception (LNG-IUC) may be better than oral contraceptive pills or depot medroxyprogesterone acetate (DMPA).
- I found some postmenopausal women were started on progesterone because of low progesterone and intended to increase sex drive. It is not necessary and also harmful.
- I also found some postmenopausal women who had hysterectomies and were started on progesterone which caused the patients unnecessary side effects like weight gain.
- Pay extra attention to what you eat and exercise daily.

What can I do if I am prescribed antihistamine medication long term?

First generation antihistamine medications or non-specific antihistamine medications are known to be associated with weight gain.

The commonly used ones are:

- Diphenhydramine (Benadryl)-commonly used for allergy and as a sleep aid.
- Cyproheptadine used to treat allergies and other conditions.

Here is what you can do:

- If you are treating an allergy, you might ask for other non-drowsy antihistamine second or third generation medication or other measures to treat your allergy.
- If you have to take these medications, you should pay extra attention to your diet and exercise.
- Ask if you are a good candidate to take medications like topiramate or Saxenda to prevent weight gain.

What can I do if I am started on a beta blocker?

Beta blockers are commonly used in modern medicine.

The following are a few commonly used beta-blockers.

- Acebutolol (Sectral)
- Atenolol (Tenormin)
- Bisoprolol (Zebeta)
- Metoprolol (Lopressor, Toprol-XL)
- Nadolol (Corgard)
- Nebivolol (Bystolic)
- Propranolol (Inderal LA, InnoPran XL)

Here is what you can do:

- If you are prescribed a beta blocker for high blood pressure, ask your doctor if it's possible to use other high blood pressure medications.

- If you are prescribed a beta blocker for migraine prophylaxis, you can also ask your doctor if you can use other medications instead.
- If you are prescribed a beta blocker for heart failure or heart protection, then you might have to take it. Pay more attention to what you eat and exercise.
- If you happen to have diabetes, ask your doctor if you are qualified to use GLP-1 agonist or SGLT2 antagonist.
- Ask your doctor if you are qualified for weight loss medication like topiramate or Saxenda.

Chapter 22. A Few Conditions Need to Be Excluded

What is hypothyroidism?

Thyroid hormone affects every cell, every tissue, every organ in our body. Without it, our body cannot function properly. If hypothyroidism is not properly treated, it can cause obesity and an array of problems.

For details, please refer to my book ***"Hashimoto's thyroiditis, Hypothyroidism Fatigue".*** It is available on Amazon.com.

What is polycystic ovarian syndrome?

Polycystic ovary syndrome (PCOS) is the most common endocrine disorder in women during their reproductive ages. It is primarily characterized by ovulatory dysfunction leading to very irregular menstrual periods and infertility and over production of the male hormone (hyperandrogenism) associated with abnormal hair growth and excessive acne.

It has been associated with a plethora of cardiometabolic consequences, with obesity, insulin resistance, prediabetes, diabetes, fatty liver, hypertension, blood clot, cancer and et al.

Statistically 50-90% of PCOS patients are obese and have difficulties in losing weight.

Does polycystic ovarian syndrome cause obesity?

I think it dose. However, in the scientific community, this is still controversial, since we still do not know the mechanism causing obesity and we still do not know which came first, "the chicken or the egg".

What is Cushing's syndrome?

Endogenous Cushing's syndrome is caused by excessive production of cortisol from the adrenal gland (pituitary tumor or adrenal tumor). It is relatively uncommon but is a very serious condition. We cannot afford to miss although sometimes it is very difficult to make the diagnosis. Cushing's syndrome can also be caused by use of steroids like long term use of prednisone for other conditions.

What is the feature of obesity in Cushing's syndrome?

The first characteristic is moon face. Fat accumulation in the cheeks results in a "moon" face and facial rounding.

The second characteristic is "buffalo hump". "Buffalo hump" or dorsocervical fat pad is common and is usually consistent with the general degree of obesity.

The third characteristic is filled supraclavicular fossae. Enlarged fat pads that fill the supraclavicular fossae and obscure the clavicles are one of the most specific signs of Cushing's syndrome. However, I found it is pretty common in the general population with obesity.

The fourth characteristic is the progressive nature of obesity, but usually the patient dose not extreme obesity.

What is male hypogonadism?

Simply to say it is low "T". Low "T" can cause obesity, and the treatment of low "T" increases leanness and reduces fatness. However, obesity can cause low "T". This is another "chicken and egg" problem.

What is growth hormone deficiency?

Growth hormone deficiency increases visceral fat (most inside of the abdomen). Children with growth hormone deficiency treated with growth hormone reduce fatness significantly.

What is hypothalamic obesity?

The hypothalamus governs metabolism and satiety. In animals, obesity can be induced by injury to the ventromedial or paraventricular region of the hypothalamus or the amygdala.

I have a few patients who had brain surgery for craniopharyngioma and rapidly developed obesity and fatty liver.

Why can some intraabdominal benign tumors be confused with obesity?

We make the diagnosis of obesity by weight (BMI) and abdominal circumference.

Some intraabdominal tumors, especially benign ovarian tumors grow very slow and insidiously. If obesity is present to start with, it is very difficult to find via a simple physical examination. I saw a report of a 132-pound ovarian tumor that was removed from a young woman in 2018. I have found a 20-pound ovarian tumor in a patient.

I order abdominal ultrasounds often for several reasons. I use it to make patients aware that they already have fatty liver which is the number one cause for cirrhosis in America. If I suspect the fatness is not matching the weight, I recommend an abdominal ultrasound to make sure there is no intraabdominal tumor.

What is the single gene mutation causing obesity?

There are a few conditions caused by a single gene mutation leading to obesity. In reality, they are very rare. We should not do extensive testing for them except in highly suspected cases.

What is leptin?

Leptin is produced in fat cells and tells the brain how much fat is in the body. If you have more fat, you will have more leptin. Then it signals brain centers to reduce the energy intake.

The mouse model of leptin function has been established. The Ob/Ob mice have the leptin gene mutation. They can grow 3-4 times larger and can be treated with leptin.

The db/db rats have diabetes and obesity. They have leptin receptor mutation.

There are some human cases of leptin or leptin receptor mutation, but they are very rare.

When should we suspect leptin related obesity?

If you have the following, we need to be alerted.

- You are the product of consanguinity (your parents are related by blood).
- You have an insatiable appetite. Your family member has to lock the refrigerator, otherwise, you will eat until you vomit.
- Your obesity started at infancy/early childhood.
- Otherwise, you are pretty normal.

What is melanocortin-4 receptor?

The leptin anorectic effect is believed through the melanocortin-4 receptor. It is believed that the mutation of melanocortin-4 receptor is much more common. The patients are similar to leptin related obesity but taller than average.

What is proopiomelanocortin (POMC) deficiency?

POMC is a precursor for ACTH and melanocyte-stimulating hormone. The ACTH is important for cortisol secretion. The melanocyte-stimulating hormone is important for melanin production (through melanocortin receptor-1) and also the ligand for melanocortin-4 receptor suppressing appetite.

The POMC deficiency can cause early obesity. These patients also have other problems like adrenal insufficiency crisis and red hair.

Successfully treated cases have been reported.

What is PCSK-1?

PCSK-1, prohormone convertase 1/3 (PC1/3), was one of the first genes linked to single gene early-onset obesity. PC1/3 is the enzyme to activate other protease involved in the processing of a variety of neuropeptides and prohormones in endocrine tissues. PC1/3 activity is essential for the activating cleavage of many peptide hormone precursors implicated in the regulation of food ingestion, glucose homeostasis, and energy homeostasis, for example, proopiomelanocortin, proinsulin, proglucagon, and proghrelin.

What is Prader-Willi syndrome?

The Prader-Willi syndrome is a neurodegenerative disorder that is caused by genetic abnormalities of the long arm of chromosome 15 (q11-13).

When should we suspect Prader-Willi syndrome?

- If you were born with weak muscle tone and poor feeding, your voracious appetite developed later.
- Besides obesity, you might have an array of other issues like short stature, behavior problems (irritability, tantrums), delayed development, delayed sexual development. You might see an endocrinologist like me for short stature and/sexual development.
- Your doctor might give you the diagnosis already since you have special facial features: almond-shaped eyes, narrow bridge of nose, narrowing of forehead at the temples, thin upper lip, and upturned mouth.

Should I have genetic testing?

More and more genes will be found to be related to obesity. The reality is the genes favoring fat storage are passed down from our ancestry. The majority of obesity is caused by many genes and interaction of our environment. Unless you have any of the above specific high suspicious factors, you do not need genetic testing.

Chapter 23. Weight Loss Medications

Why do you recommend weight loss medications?

Weight loss medication is never the first line of therapy. I coach people to lose weight by lifestyle changes and stress management. However, weight loss is like everything else, easy to say and hard to do. It is extremely hard in dealing with eating. We are wired to eat as much as we can and do as little as we can. We want to save energy. This is in our genes.

I prescribe weight loss medications for the following reasons:

- If used properly they work.
- Eating is a habit and changing the habit to form a new habit takes time. Using medication helps people to form a new way of eating.
- Boosts the weight loss, and sometimes it can boost people's courage and confidence and encourage them to do more.
- Some medication can also increase energy level and mental concentration.

What are the FDA approved medications on the market?

Currently we have the following medications FDA approved for the sole purpose of weight loss. All weight loss medications are contraindicated if you are **pregnant or breastfeeding.**

- Orlistat works through inhibiting fat digestion. It has benefits with regard to glycemia, lipids, and blood pressure; long-duration trials; and safety profile.
- Saxenda. Saxenda is liraglutide which is a GLP-1 agonist (for more information, please read my diabetes book). It increases satiety , inhibits appetite and slows gastric empty. Liraglutide is a daily injection and is also used for treating diabetes.
- Belviq is lorcaserin which can be used in obese patients with diabetes, hypertension, and/or dyslipidemia.

- Sympathomimetic drugs (stimulants) like phentermine, benzphetamine, phendimetrazine, and diethylpropion. Clinically they are only US Food and Drug Administration (FDA) approved for short-term use, have more side effects, and there is potential for abuse. I use a low dose of phentermine often.
- Combinations like Qsymia (phentermine-topiramate) (extended release). It may have more side effects and be more effective.
- Combinations like Contrave (bupropion-naltrexone) (sustained release). I do not use often because in my experience, it does not work very well and most of my patients are using SSRI (anti-depression medication). The use of SSRI increases the risks of Contrave.

- Plenity, hydrogel pill as a weight loss device, has been approved for weight loss in April 2019 and will be available in 2020.

What is orlistat?

Fat needs lipase (an enzyme) to digest in order to be absorbed. Orlistat is a lipase inhibitor. it can inhibit around 30% fat digestion.

Can I buy orlistat over the counter (OTC)?

You can buy orlistat OTC by the name of Alli.

Alli: OTC labeling: 60 mg three times daily with each main meal containing fat (maximum dose: 180 mg/day). You do not need to take it if you eat a meal without fat. It is also okay to miss a dose. 90 capsules cost around $45-50.

What is the prescription version of orlistat?

Xenical: 120 mg three times daily with each main meal containing fat (during or up to one hour after the meal); omit dose if meal is occasionally missed or contains no fat. The list price for Xenical is $600-700 for 90 capsules. Most insurance does not pay for this. Therefore, I just recommend patients to get the OTC Alli which is cheaper.

What should I know before I start orlistat?

Before you start orlistat, you need to know the following:

- Severe and common gastrointestinal side effects: Oily rectal leakage (4% to 27%), abdominal distress (≤26%), abdominal pain (≤26%), flatulence with discharge (2% to 24%), bowel urgency (3% to 22%), steatorrhea (6% to 20%), oily evacuation (2% to 12%), frequent bowel movements (3% to 11%), nausea (4% to 8%), fecal incontinence (2% to 8%), infectious diarrhea (≤5%), rectal pain (3% to 5%), gingival disease (4%), cholelithiasis (3%), abdominal distension (in patients with diabetes).

- Gallstones (cholelithiasis): Substantial weight loss may increase the risk of gallstones.
- Liver damage (hepatotoxicity): Cases of severe liver injury (some fatal) with hepatocellular necrosis or acute hepatic failure have been reported; liver transplantation has been required in some patients. You need to call your doctor or go to the ER and stop the treatment if you have no appetite (anorexia), itching (pruritus), yellow skin/eyes (jaundice), dark urine, light colored stools or right upper quadrant pain.
- Kidney stone: Increased levels of urinary oxalate following treatment may occur in some patients. Oxalate and calcium forms kidney stones. Cases of kidney stones (oxalate nephrolithiasis) and kidney disease (oxalate nephropathy) with renal failure have been reported. Monitor renal function in patients at risk for renal impairment; use with caution in patients with a history of high urine oxalate (hyperoxaluria) or calcium oxalate kidney stones.
- This is the OTC medication. This doesn't mean you do not need to talk to your doctor before you start it.

To what major drug interactions do I need to pay attention?

Amiodarone: This is the common medication cardiologists use to treat irregular heart beat like atrial fibrillation. Orlistat may decrease the serum concentration of amiodarone. Your doctor should check your amiodarone level and monitor its effectiveness.

Propafenone: Propafenone is the medication cardiologists use to replace amiodarone for less side effects. Orlistat may decrease the serum concentration of propafenone.

Anticonvulsants: Orlistat may decrease the serum concentration of anticonvulsants.

Exceptions: Fosphenytoin; Pentobarbital; Thiopental.

Antiretroviral Agents: Orlistat may decrease the serum concentration of antiretroviral agents.

Cyclosporine (Systemic): Cyclosporine is an anti-rejection medication. Orlistat may decrease the serum concentration of cyclosporine (systemic). Management: Administer orlistat at least three hours before or after oral cyclosporine. Remember, you need to take three hours apart from other medication.

Levothyroxine: Orlistat may decrease the serum concentration of levothyroxine. Management: Separate administration of oral levothyroxine and orlistat by at least four hours. Monitor patients closely for signs and symptoms of hypothyroidism.

Multivitamins/Fluoride/minerals: Orlistat may decrease the serum concentration of multivitamins/fluoride. Specifically, orlistat may impair absorption of fat-soluble vitamins like A, D, E, K. Take multiple vitamins at 3-4 hours apart. You also need to take active vitamin D like calcitriol, paricalcitol three to four hours apart. I recommend omitting the dose if you are taking multivitamins or active vitamin D.

Coumadin (vitamin K antagonists): Orlistat may enhance the anticoagulant effect of coumadin which might cause severe bleeding. You need to let your doctor know so your labs can be monitored more closely.

What is Saxenda?

Saxenda is liraglutide which is a GLP-1 agonist. Liraglutide is commonly used for managing diabetes. Saxenda is prescribed for weight loss for those patients without diabetes. For patients with diabetes, I usually use liraglutide. The trade name is Victoza. The maximum dose for Victoza is 1.8 mg daily, while the maximum dose for Saxenda is 3 mg daily. Both are injectable with very good effects. Unfortunately, most insurance doesn't cover either for weight loss. If you have diabetes, most insurance will cover Victoza.

How do you prescribe Victoza or Saxenda?

Sample prescription for Victoza: Victoza one box (carton) with two refills, **Usage**: 1.8 mg sc once daily in the morning.

I usually prescribe one box (carton) for one month which has three pens inside. I ask my patient for the first week to start 0.6 mg sc once daily in the morning, and then increase to 1.2 mg once daily the next week. If possible, increase to 1.8 mg sc once daily in the morning the third week.

Sample prescription for Saxenda: Saxenda one box (carton) with two refills. Usage: 3 mg sc once daily in the morning.

I usually prescribe 1 box (carton) for one month which has 5 pens inside. I ask my patient first week to start 0.6 mg sc once daily in the morning, and then increase to 1.2 mg once daily the next week, and then increase by 0.6 mg the third week if possible. The maximum dose is 3 mg once daily.

What do I need to pay attention to before I start Victoza/Saxenda?

Again, I have to emphasize that Victoza is not licensed to treat obesity alone. It is licensed to treat diabetes. You need to pay attention to the common warnings for all weight loss medications. You need to pay attention to the following:

- If you have a personal or family history of pancreatitis, pancreatic neoplasms or cancer, you should not take them.
- Family history of a rare thyroid cancer like medullary thyroid cancer or multiple endocrine neoplasia 2A or 2B.
- It is very rare, but it has been reported that this group of medications, like other medications, might cause hypersensitivity which can be life threatening.
- If you have a very weak immune system and easily get all sorts of infections, discuss this with your prescribing physician.
- Victoza/Saxenda slows gastric emptying. It might affect other medications absorption. You need to let your doctor know all the medications you are taking. If you are taking some medications which need rapid absorption or need peak concentration to take effect (like some antibiotics), you might not be able to take it.
- Victoza/Saxenda can be put on hold if you are severely ill. For example, if you have a fever, severe nausea, vomiting, and dehydration, remember, it is okay to discontinue on occasions.
- If you have a diagnosis of gastroparesis, you should not take them unless you specifically discuss this with your treating physician. These medications might cause your gastroparesis to manifest more symptomatic.
- Victoza/Saxenda are not insulin, but if you are using them with insulin or sulfonylurea or insulin releasing agents like glipizide, glimepiride or glyburide or glinides like Starlix, they can cause low sugar

(hypoglycemia). Therefore, the dose of insulin or sulfonylureas or glinides might need to be adjusted.

- If you do not think it has worked for you, you should stop using it in one-two months.

To what major drug interaction do I need to pay attention?

The major concern is the slower gastric emptying. If you think you have severe gastroparesis, I recommend to not use it, since all other oral medications theoretically can be affected. As some medication requires a peak drug level to work, you need a medication to be absorbed faster to reach the peak level. Even for medications like thyroid medication, if you have severe gastroparesis, the absorption can be delayed and hindered.

What is Belviq?

Belviq is lorcaserin which is a serotonin 2C receptor agonist. It is an appetite suppressant. A recent large clinic trial (2018) revealed that Belviq is safe and effective for cardiovascular disease risk. It also reduces blood pressure, blood sugar and "bad cholesterol" LDL.

What do I need to know before I start Belviq?

Besides needing to pay attention to the common warnings for all weight loss medication, you need to pay attention to the following:

- You should not use it if you are on any sort of anti-depression medications.
- If you are on some sort of anti-nausea medications chronically.
- If have heart valvular disease.
- If you have severe liver dysfunction, or if your kidneys are not working well (eGFR<30).
- CNS depression: May cause confusion, somnolence, fatigue, and cognitive impairment (difficulty with concentration/attention/ memory); patients must be cautioned about performing tasks which require mental alertness (e.g., operating machinery or driving).
- It might cause prolactin to increase which can cause breast secretion (galactorrhea), breast enlargement (gynecomastia) or low sex hormones.
- Persistent erection (priapism): May occur with use; men with erections lasting more than four hours should immediately discontinue

lorcaserin and seek emergency medical attention to avoid irreversible damage to erectile tissue.

- Do not use in a patient with a diagnosis of pulmonary hypertension.
- If overdosed, it can cause euphoria. Hallucinations and dissociation have been observed with lorcaserin at supratherapeutic doses.
- If you have diabetes, make sure to adjust your diabetes medication, otherwise your risk for low sugar is increased.
- It is a moderate inhibitor of CYP2D6 (liver metabolism enzyme). Lots of medications are metabolized through CYP2D6. If you are taking many other medications, be sure to ask your pharmacist to run a drug-drug interaction screening.

How do you prescribe Belviq?

Belviq has 10 mg immediate release tablets and extended release Belviq XR 20 mg tablets. I usually prescribe extended release only.

Sample Prescription: Belviq XR 20 mg 30 tablets no refills. Usage: once daily in the morning.

There are two versions: immediate release 10 mg tablets or extended release 20 mg tablets. I always prescribe extended release for the convenience. The medication can be taken with or without food. I recommend taking it in the early morning. If no weight loss occurs after one-month usage, I would stop it. Patients do better if working with a doctor for weight loss. This medication also has extensive drug interaction. You want to make sure the patient is not being started on other medications in between visits.

Your prescribing physician needs to be REMS trained. A Risk Evaluation and Mitigation Strategy (REMS) is a drug safety program set by FDA for some high-risk medication.

What are sympathomimetic drugs for weight loss?

They are stimulants like phentermine, benzphetamine, phendimetrazine, and diethylpropion.

I usually only use phentermine because it is affordable, and I have more experience with it.

What do I need to know before I start phentermine?

Contraindicated for the following conditions:

- Hypersensitivity or idiosyncrasy to phentermine, other sympathomimetic amines or any component of the formulation;
- History of cardiovascular disease (e.g., arrhythmias, heart failure, coronary artery disease, stroke, uncontrolled hypertension);
- Overactive thyroid (hyperthyroidism); glaucoma; agitated states;
- History of drug abuse; used during or within 14 days following MAO inhibitor therapy (a kind of antidepressant medication);
- Pregnancy or breastfeeding;
- Tourette's syndrome.

Major potential side effects:

- Central Nervous System: Very interesting, since some people reported having depression. In the prescription notes it says it might cause physical impairment. This needs to be watched. Most of my people report having more energy and being more focused, getting more things done. Some patients have anxiety, insomnia. **Alcohol makes it much worse. Do not drink alcohol.**
- Cardiovascular System: it can cause palpitations, or irregular heartbeat. It might be related to heart failure or heart attack.
- Primary pulmonary hypertension (PPH): A rare, frequently fatal disease of the lungs. It causes shortness of breath, lower extremity swelling and so on. It is difficult to differentiate clinically from regular heart failure. It requires an ultrasound or catheterization to make the diagnosis.
- Valvular heart disease: Serious regurgitant cardiac valvular disease has been reported to occur in patients receiving a combination of phentermine and fenfluramine (not used in USA anymore) or dexfenfluramine (not used in USA anymore). The possibility of an association between valvular heart disease and the use of phentermine alone cannot be ruled out.

What are the formulations of phentermine?

Brand Names:

- Adipex-P, 37.5 mg/capsule or tablet.
- Lomaira, 8 mg/tablet.

Adipex-P has a generic version which is 1/15 price of brand name Adipex-P.

Sample prescription: Phentermine 37.5 mg x30 tablet, no refills. **Usage**: take ½ tab orally every day in the morning.

I only prescribe 30-tab one time (state law requirement). I also only prescribe tablets since I need them to cut. My maximum dose is half tab daily. You can take it at any time with or without food. However, try not to take at the end of the day since it might cause a sleep problem. Do not use on patients with stage IV, V renal failure.

Sample prescription: Lomaira 8 mg x 90, no refills. Usage: take orally one tab three times a day.

I usually do not prescribe Lomaira because it is a brand name and very expensive. I only prescribe it because my patient needs a lower dose than phentermine. I have some patients who only need to take one tab in the morning.

Generic phentermine is a tiny pill. If a patient wants to save money, I just prescribe generic phentermine to be cut into quarters.

To what major drug interactions do I need to pay attention?

Phentermine is like lorcaserin which has lots of drug interactions. Every visit, we need to check your new medication. Therefore, it is very important to visit your doctor and report your new medications.

- Acebrophylline/doxofylline: it is a bronchodilator for asthma or COPD. May enhance the stimulatory effect of CNS Stimulants.
- Alcohol: It may enhance the adverse/toxic effect of phentermine. Therefore, do not drink alcohol.
- Ascorbic Acid: May decrease the serum concentration of phentermine. Do not take vitamin C.
- ADHD medications. May enhance the hypertensive effect of phentermine. I do **not** use them together. If you are taking one of the following medications, you should let your doctor know.

  Commonly used medications are:
  - Amphetamines
    - Adderall XR (generic-dextroamphetamine/amphetamine)

    - Dexedrine (generic - dextroamphetamine)
    - Dyanavel XR
    - Evekeo
    - Procentra (generic - dextroamphetamine)
    - Vyvanse
  - Methamphetamine (Desoxyn)
  - Methylphenidate. The brand names are:
    - Aptensio XR
    - Metadate ER
    - Concerta (generic available)
    - Daytrana
    - Ritalin (generic available)
    - Ritalin LA (generic available)
    - Methylin (generic available)
    - Quillichew
    - Quillivant
    - Focalin (generic available)
  - Atomoxetine (Strattera)
- Bupropion: May enhance the neuroexcitatory and/or seizure-potentiating effect of agents in patients with seizures.
- Carbonic Anhydrase Inhibitors: May decrease the excretion of amphetamines. Exceptions: Brinzolamide; Dorzolamide. Monitor therapy.
- CYP2D6 Inhibitors (Strong): May increase the serum concentration of Amphetamines. Monitor therapy. Commonly used medications are:
  - Certain anti-depression medications: fluoxetine, paroxetine, bupropion.
  - Cinacalcet (for hyperparathyroidism).
  - Ritonavir (antivirus medication)
- Guanethidine: May enhance the arrhythmogenic effect of Sympathomimetics. Guanethidine may enhance the hypertensive effect of sympathomimetics. Monitor therapy.
- Multivitamins/Fluoride: May decrease the serum concentration of amphetamines. More specifically, the ascorbic acid (vitamin C) in many multivitamins may decrease amphetamine concentrations.

There are more medications which have drug interactions with phentermine. You can launch a drug interaction program and have an examination.

What is Qsymia?

Qsymia is a combination of phentermine and extended-release topiramate (in one capsule). FDA approved in 2012 for long term use in management of obesity. Topiramate is an anti-seizure medication. Sometimes it is also used for migraine prophylaxis. It reduces appetite significantly and leads to weight loss.

What do I need to know before I start Qsymia?

Qsymia has two medications phentermine and topiramate. So you need to look at both medications' precautions.

Refer to the question above for phentermine.

For Topiramate, you need to pay attention to the following:

- Metabolic acidosis: may be due to reduced bicarbonate production or increased loss.
- Too high body temperature (hyperthermia) / no sweets (oligohidrosis). You need to pay attention especially when you are doing high intensity exercise.
- Vision effect. You need to pay attention if you develop acute onset of decreased visual acuity and/or eye pain. You might develop acute nearsightedness or glaucoma. You need to stop the medication immediately and see your ophthalmologist.
- Kidney stones (renal calculus/lithiasis): Consider avoiding use in patients on a ketogenic diet. The risk of kidney stones may be reduced by increasing fluid intake.
- Suicidal ideation: Pooled analysis of trials involving various antiepileptics (regardless of indication) showed an increased risk of suicidal thoughts/behavior (incidence rate: 0.43% treated patients compared to 0.24% of patients receiving placebo).

To what major common drug interaction do I need to pay attention?

Read the above drug interactions of phentermine.

For topiramate, pay attention to the following major common drug interactions:

- Amitriptyline: Topiramate may enhance the central nervous system depressant effect of amitriptyline. Topiramate may increase serum concentrations of the active metabolite(s) of amitriptyline. Topiramate may increase the serum concentration of amitriptyline.

- Azelastine (Nasal): Topiramate may enhance the central nervous system depressant effect of Azelastine. Azelastine is used to treat hay fever and allergy symptoms including runny nose, sneezing, and itchy nose.
- Hormones or oral contraceptives. Topiramate might reduce the effect. Contraceptive failure is possible.
- Lithium: Topiramate may increase the serum concentration of lithium. I recommend monitoring the lithium level. Lithium can cause lots of adverse effects on the thyroid and kidneys.
- Orlistat: It reduces the absorption of medications like topiramate.
- Thiazide and thiazide-like diuretics: May enhance the low potassium (hypokalemic) effect of topiramate. Thiazide and Thiazide-like diuretics may increase the serum concentration of topiramate. Management: Monitor for increased topiramate levels/adverse effects (e.g., low potassium) with initiation/dose increase of a thiazide diuretic. Closely monitor serum potassium.
- Zolpidem: it is a sleep medicine. Both drugs central nervous system's depressant effects may be enhanced. The dose of zolpidem might need to be reduced.

What are the formulations of Qsymia?

Capsule, extended release, oral:

Qsymia: 3.75/23: Phentermine 3.75 mg [immediate release] and topiramate 23 mg [extended release] [contains tartrazine]

Qsymia: 7.5/46: Phentermine 7.5 mg [immediate release] and topiramate 46 mg [extended release] [contains tartrazine]

Qsymia: 11.25/69: Phentermine 11.25 mg [immediate release] and topiramate 69 mg [extended release] [contains tartrazine]

Qsymia: 15/92: Phentermine 15 mg [immediate release] and topiramate 92 mg [extended release] [contains tartrazine]

How is Qsymia prescribed?

Initiation: need two prescriptions.

- First two weeks. Qsymia 3.75/23 x 14 capsules, no refills. Usage: one capsule orally daily in the morning.
- Thereafter: Qsymia 7.5/46 x30 capsules, no refills. Usage: one capsule orally daily in the morning.

Comments: it is recommended to continue for three months and if the weight loss < 3%, increase to the next dose level. I usually let my patients try for one month on the dose of 7.5/46. If the weight loss <4 lbs for the month and if the patient does not think it affects his or her appetite, I would increase to the next dose level.

The high dose level prescription:

- Qsymia 11.25/69 x 14 capsules, no refills. Usage. Take one capsule orally daily in the morning.
- Thereafter: Qsymia 15/92 x 30 capsules, no refills. Usage: take one capsule orally daily in the morning.

Comments: it is recommended to continue for three months and if the weight loss <3%, then stop the treatment. I usually let my patients try one month. If the weight loss <4 lbs for the month and if the patient does not think it affects his or her appetite, I would stop it.

In 2012 and early 2013 I wrote quite a few prescriptions because everyone was excited. The company also provided some coupons. However, the weight loss was not much better than phentermine alone in my experience and it is so much more expensive. Most people cannot tolerate the price. No one was able to continue. Now, I barely use it.

Can I go to a compound pharmacy to make the combination?

Theoretically, you can. As a matter of fact, a local compounding pharmacy approached me to send patients to them. But I did not trust them. As you know, this medication is a controlled substance and the dose error can cause severe if not deadly consequences.

Can I ask my doctor to prescribe phentermine and topiramate separately?

Theoretically you can, but I have never done that and I am not planning to do that.

Can I just take topiramate for weight loss?

If you want to ask your doctor for that, you need to understand it is off-label use (not FDA approved).

Antipsychotic-induced weight gain (off-label use): Oral initial dose of 25 mg twice daily for one week; continue to increase in increments of 25 to 50 mg each week based on response and tolerability up to 300 mg/day. Target doses in clinical trials ranged from 100 to 300 mg/day.

What is Contrave?

Contrave is the combination of bupropion and naltrexone which was approved by the FDA in September 2014 as an adjunct to diet and exercise in patients with BMI ≥30 kg/m2 or ≥27 kg/m2 in the presence of at least one weight-related comorbidity. Bupropion is an anti-depression medication. Naltrexone is an opioid-receptor antagonist used to treat alcohol and opioid dependence.

What do I need to know before I start?

Do not use Contrave if you have one of the following:

- Hypersensitivity to bupropion, naltrexone, or any other component of the formulation;
- Concomitant use of other bupropion-containing products (e.g., including but not limited to Wellbutrin, Wellbutrin SR, Wellbutrin XL, Aplenzin, Zyban);
- Chronic opioid, opiate agonist (e.g., methadone) or partial agonist (e.g., buprenorphine) use;
- Acute opioid withdrawal;
- Uncontrolled hypertension; recent heart attack or stroke;
- Seizure disorder or a history of seizures;
- Bulimia or anorexia nervosa; abrupt discontinuation of alcohol, benzodiazepines, barbiturates, and antiepileptic drugs;
- Concomitant use of MAOIs (concurrently or within 14 days of discontinuing the MAOI or naltrexone/bupropion); MAOIs are monoamine oxidase inhibitors which are the first group of medications developed for depression.

- Younger than 24 years old because the risk for suicide might be increased;
- Severe liver dysfunction;
- Severe renal dysfunction;
- Patients with glaucoma;
- You should not drink alcohol if taking this medication.

How to prescribe Contrave?

Contrave 8/90 120 tabs, one refill. Usage: as directed.

Initiation:

Week 1: One tablet (naltrexone 8 mg/bupropion 90 mg) once daily in the morning.

Week 2: Increase to one tablet twice daily administered in the morning and evening.

Week 3: Increase to two tablets in the morning and 1 tablet in the evening.

Week 4: Increase to two tablets twice daily administered in the morning and evening and continue for the remainder of the treatment course.

Comments:

I used this medication when it was initially available. I found that the medication was not really very effective and quite expensive, too, although you can get a month's supply from Contrave.com for $99. It is still a lot of money for my patients. Also, the cardiovascular safety trial was discontinued, and the safety is not very clear. I use it on really selective patients.

Concomitant use with CYP2B6 inhibitors (eg, ticlopidine, clopidogrel): Maximum dose: one tablet (naltrexone 8 mg/bupropion 90 mg) twice daily.

What is Plenity?

The FDA approved an oral hydrogel capsule that induces feeling of fullness. The capsules release thousands of non-aggregating particles that rapidly absorb water in the stomach, creating small individual gel pieces to make you feel full but without calories. It is for adults with a BMI over 25 kg/m^{2}. with or without complications. The hydrogel capsule contains cellulose, citric acid, sodium stearyl fumarate, gelatin and titanium oxide. If you have allergy or over sensitive to these substances, you should not take it.

I like this concept. Portion control is crucial in weight loss. Many patients cannot do it because they feel not full and starving all the time. I think it will help diabetes and fatty liver also. Based on FDA documents, it seems very effective and the side effects are limited. It might affect other medication absorption. I am looking forward to prescribing it when it is available in 2020.

Similar idea is the gastric balloon. However, it needs gastroenterologist to put it in and retrieve from your stomach. It increases the cost.

Chapter 24. Common Dietary Supplements for Weight Loss

Do you recommend any dietary supplements for your patients?

NO, I do not recommend any dietary supplements for my patients for weight loss. I am asked this question by my patients all the time. Here are the reasons that I do not recommend any supplements for weight loss:

- The effectiveness has not been well established. Most ads are overstated.
- Some stimulants might have some effectiveness; however, safety is a concern.
- What you can buy OTC does not mean it's safe or effective.
- What is natural does not mean safe. Even if something can help weight loss that does not mean you should use it. Cocaine is natural and can cause weight loss. We all know we should not use cocaine.
- Sometimes, the OTC medication can cause a drug interaction with prescription medications, like St. John's Wort.
- I want my patients to realize there is no magic pill yet in terms of weight loss. The fat has to be "burned" and breathed out as carbon dioxide and part of it becomes water. Small amounts of ketones can also be lost from urine.
- They are not cheap either. These can be a big financial burden to patients.
- However, I do recommend Shirataki noodles for meal replacement but not as a supplement.

What are the main supplements which are marketed to increase one's energy expenditure?

Ephedra Sinica - Ma Huang in Chinese, is the most popular. The effective component is ephedrine, similar to adrenaline. In Chinese medicine, it is used for asthma or bronchitis. Bitter orange and country mallow contain related chemicals. In 2004, the U.S. Food and Drug Administration (FDA) banned the sale of supplements containing ephedrine.

You actually can buy Ma Huang tea legally in US.

Another commonly used product for increasing energy expenditure is caffeine.

Does Ma Huang really help you lose weight?

I have not seen really good double-blind, randomized, placebo-controlled large clinical trials, but theoretically Ma Huang can help you lose weight. The active ingredient is ephedrine which is like amphetamine or adrenaline. These chemicals and hormones increase your metabolism and suppress your appetite.

What do I need to know before starting to drink Ma Huang Tea?

You need to know the following before you start:

- Ma Huang tea is just like adrenaline which increases your risk for elevated blood pressure, heart attack, and stroke. Everyone has a certain risk. You need to keep this in mind.
- Closely monitor your blood pressure. If your blood pressure has not been well controlled, do not start Ma Huang tea.
- If you have anxiety, do not drink Ma Huang Tea. It can increase your anxiety.
- Do not drink it in the afternoon or evening, since it might disturb your sleep.
- It might affect some hormone lab tests.
- If you are involved in a competitive sport, you should not use it since it will be shown in the drug test.

You should pay attention to the same items if you are using caffeine. Do not use both together.

What are the supplements proposed to increase carbohydrate metabolism?

Chromium deficiency is reported to cause insulin resistance and hyperglycemia. This is the reason people believe that the supplement of chromium might increase carbohydrate metabolism and cause weight loss.

However, clinical trials were not able to show the effect of weight loss.

There are case reports showing severe side effects from overdosing. There are case reports of rhabdomyolysis (muscle dissolved), or acute renal failure.

The common supplement is chromium picolinate in daily dosages of 200 to 400 mcg.

Ginseng is also believed to increase carbohydrate metabolism. However, there are no good clinical trials showing that. If you take too much, it can increase your blood pressure and heart rate also.

What are the supplements proposed to increase fat oxidation?

Green tea is believed to increase fat oxidation and lead to weight loss. Green tea is also a stimulant. You need to be cautious if you use other stimulants.

Licorice containing products are also believed to increase fat oxidation to reduce fat mass. However, licorice is notorious for causing hypertension and low potassium.

Pyruvate is a metabolite of glucose. Some people believe the supplement pyruvate increases fat oxidation. To me, it is really odd. Taking the metabolite of glucose is like taking sugar. I read a comprehensive review of the use of pyruvate on weight loss. The conclusion is that it does not work. My recommendation is not to take it.

Pantothenic acid (vitamin B5) is used in the synthesis of coenzyme A (CoA). CoA is used in fat, protein, and sugar metabolism. This is why people think pantothenic acid might work. Most people are not deficient of pantothenic acids, so there is no reason to think this will help you lose weight.

L-carnitine was isolated in meat more than 100 years ago and people are trying to find the function. Until 1958, it was found to facilitate long chain fatty acid to move into the mitochondria to oxidize. L-carnitine was also found to regulate glucose metabolism. This is why L-carnitine is suggested for weight loss.

I did find some clinical research showing weight loss by taking L-carnitine. However, a meta-analysis revealed that non-obese people actually lost more weight taking L-carnitine compared to obese people taking L-carnitine, 1.75 kg vs 1.25 kg. When people take L-carnitine longer the weight loss is less. What I take from these studies is that if you have L-carnitine deficiency, then it might boost your metabolism and help you lose weight, however, after some time and you are not deficient any more, it doesn't help.
It is not risk free if you take a high amount long term. New research has shown that L-carnitine is converted to trimethylamine (TMA) by the gut bacteria and converted to trimethylamine-N-oxide (TMAO) in the liver. TMAO is linked to the cause of heart attack and strokes.

High doses of L-carnitine are also linked to insulin resistance which is not good either.

L-carnitine is also shown to block thyroid hormone which is very important for cell metabolism.

So, **my recommendation** is that if you are a long-term vegetarian, it may be okay to take some L-carnitine as a supplement for a short time. If you are a meat eater, you already have more than enough. If you take more, it might cause harmful effects.

What supplements are suggested to inhibit fat formation?

Garcinia extract (Hydroxycitric acid) is believed to inhibit citrate lyase and therefore it inhibits fat synthesis. Hydroxycitric acid is derived from the Malabar tamarind tropical fruit (Garcinia cambogia) native to India. There are clinical trials showing that garcinia extract helps short term weight loss. However, there are twice as many patients who have nausea, upset stomach.

We do not know if the weight loss is coming from eating less or truly from inhibiting fat formation.

My **recommendation** is that if you are healthy and don't take excessive amounts, for a short term, it may be safe.

What supplements are proposed to inhibit fat absorption?

Chitosan, derived from chitin found in crustacean shells, is a positively charged polymer thought to prevent fat absorption by binding negatively charged fat molecules within the intestinal lumen. However, the use of chitosan does not really increase the fat excretion in healthy people. It most likely does not really work as it is supposed to. It seems well tolerated, however.

My recommendation is that since it really does not work, why take it.

What are other common products on the market for weight loss?

Dandelion appears to have diuretic activity. It causes weight loss by losing more water. I think you should not take it.

Cascara sagrada is a shrub. The dried bark is used in laxatives. Now in the US, it is sold as a dietary supplement. The long-term safety is a concern. This is why the FDA does not allow it to be sold as an OTC laxative in the US. The weight loss does not really reduce fatness. I do not recommend it for long term use. It may be safe to be used for a week.

Rhubarb is another plant in China which is used as a laxative. Some people claim it can help lose weight. The effectiveness is not clear, but if you eat it as food and do not overeat, it should be safe for short term use.

St. John's Wort is an herbaceous plant and mostly used for treating depression. Some people also believe it may help them lose weight. The effectiveness of weight loss is very limited.

St. John's Wort has many drug interactions.

There is strong evidence to suggest that St John's Wort significantly reduces the plasma concentrations of the following medicines:

- indinavir
- cyclosporin

St John's Wort may reduce the efficacy of the following medicines:

- warfarin (blood thinner)
- digoxin (mostly used for heart failure and irregular heart beat)
- theophylline (used for asthma and COPD)
- other HIV protease inhibitors (saquinavir, ritonavir, nelfinavir)
- HIV non-nucleoside reverse transcriptase inhibitors (efavirenz, nevirapine, delavirdine)
- anticonvulsants (phenytoin, carbamazepine, phenobarbitone)
- oral contraceptive pills

St. John's Wort also affects other mood medications and might cause serious side effects.

If St. John's Wort is going to be started or stopped, you need to let your doctor know that otherwise some medication might cause toxicity.

Laminaria (kelp) is a kind of seaweed. Laminaria seems to be able to form a thick, sticky gel when it comes into contact with water. It has very low carbohydrates and low calories. In many Asian countries, we eat it as food. I think the weight loss property may be due to its bulky effect. You eat a lot of laminaria and eat less of others. It is one of my favorites. However, I do not eat it all the time. It has lots of iodine. I recommend my patients with iodine deficiency to eat it. Unfortunately, most Americans are not used to it. Another concern is for renal failure patients since it has a relatively high level of potassium. My recommendation is that it is safe to eat it occasionally.

Spirulina is an algae (blue-green algae). People think it might help lose weight. It is very nutritious. Unfortunately, there are also reports that it might be contaminated by some neurotoxin.

Guggul is made from the oily sap (gum resin) of the guggul tree, which is native to India, Bangladesh, and Pakistan. It is used as an oral supplement and believed to help weight loss. It is also used for lowering cholesterol because it has a good amount of plant cholesterol. Guggul can cause an allergic reaction that sometimes can be very serious. It can also cause restlessness, apprehension, and breakdown of muscle tissue.

Apple cider vinegar is fermented crushed apple. It is a vinegar with lots of acid. I think if you use it as a condiment it is safe. The major concern for consuming too much is the low potassium which can cause cramping and more seriously can affect other medications and cause irregular heartbeats.

Shirataki noodles or Tofu are suggested to help weight loss. I believe it. Shirataki noodles are made from Glucomannan, a natural, water-soluble dietary fiber extracted from the roots of the elephant yam, also known as konjac. It has no carbs and no calories. Some people take glucomannan to lose weight. It will not work if you are still eating your regular meals. In a clinical trial the exact result was shown. There is no weight loss property if you only take glucomannan as a supplement. You need to eat it as meal replacement. You can buy it from local grocery stores or online stores.

Turmeric (Curcumin) also has effects to inhibit adipocyte differentiation and to promote antioxidant activities. The clinical trial is not concrete, but this has been used as a food condiment for thousands of years. If you do not take large quantities, I presume it is safe.

Aloe Vera Juice are also believed to help people lose weight by reduce the fat absorption and increase fat metabolism. I could not find any clinical trials to support these claims. However, it should be safe if you drink limited amount.

Bitter Melon (Gourd) is also believed to reduce blood sugar and aid people losing weight. In China, people eat it as vegetables. Chinese believe it do lots good things for your body. My parents used to love it. I never love it. It is bitter. You need to get used to it. In China, people eat in large quantity. It should be safe. If you want to try, you can buy it from Asian grocery store. Be sure to google some recipes.

Moringa leaf is from a fast-growing tree native to India and other Asia countries. Africa and South America countries also have wide present. The leaf was found to have dense nutrients like all essential amino acids, vitamins and minerals. Moringa leaf is suggested to lower blood sugar and aiding lose weight. I think this need more research. India has a higher diabetes rate than Americans now.

Fenugreek belongs to a legume family. In China, it has been used for promoting milk production for thousands of years. In India, it is used as a spice. It has high protein and high fibers. Now it is claimed to lower blood sugar and lose weight. You can buy from online or local grocery stores.

Gymnema sylvestre is called gurmar meaning "sugar destroyer". It is used to diabetes in India. It is believed to curb sweet craving, reduce sugar, reduce cholesterol and help losing weight.

Oregano is a flowering plant in the mint family. It is native to temperate Western and Southwestern Eurasia and the Mediterranean region.

Rosemary extract is also believed in enhancing the burning of sugar and blocking the formation of fat.

What are prebiotics?

Prebiotics are soluble fibers in food which cannot be digested by humans but are fermented by bacteria in the gut as food for them. They help gut flora. They are reported to help weight loss, reduce triglycerides and bad cholesterol. They are also shown to reduce inflammation in the gut and reduce fatty liver.

How can I take in more prebiotics?

You should eat more natural food. The following foods are packed with a high amount of prebiotics.

- Raw chicory root: 64.5% of dry weight.
- Jerusalem artichoke: 31.6% of dry weight.
- Raw dandelion greens:24.3% of dry weight.
- Raw garlic: 17.5% of dry weight.
- Raw leek: 9.7% of dry weight.
- Raw onion: 8.6% of dry weight.
- Cooked onion: 5% of dry weight
- Raw asparagus: 5% of dry weight

- Raw wheat bran: 5% dry weight
- Whole grain/oats:5% of weight
- Banana: 1% of weight

Each source has a different amount of prebiotic fibers. For instance, oats and barley have high amounts of beta-glucans, fruit and berries contain pectins, seeds contain gums, onions and Jerusalem artichokes are rich in inulin and oligofructose, and bananas and legumes contain resistant starch.

Can I buy prebiotics supplements? And how much should I take?

Yes, you can buy prebiotics and it is recommended to take 4-8 grams daily.

What are probiotics? And can I take them to lose weight?

Probiotics are microbiota believed to be beneficial to your health. Many species are identified. The predominates are *Lactobacillus* and/or *Bifidobacterium* species. Some reports claim that taking probiotics can help lose weight. Well to me, we need better scientific data. As far as I know, we even do not know if those commercial probiotics can survive the acid in our stomach. There are many brands. You can also obtain from food like yogurt, kefir.

Should I take both prebiotics and probiotics?

In my opinion, taking probiotics alone is useless. First, as I discussed above, we really do not know if the probiotics you are taking can or cannot survive the stomach acid and get to the place they need to go which is the large intestine. If you do not change the way you live, you still have the problem which causes you to have imbalance of gut microflora. Even if the probiotics reach the place, they cannot survive because the environment is not suitable for them to live. Let me give you an example. You want to grow some bacteria in purified water. Guess what? They will not grow because there is no nutrition. If you add some nutrition to the water, if only a few bacteria, they will multiply very quickly. Bacteria can split and double the number every two hours. In my opinion, most important is that you change your diet so your gut microflora can have food to eat and they can multiply. They multiply very fast. You really do not need to take probiotics. If you do, you need to change your diet, otherwise they are useless. The bottom-line is that if you think this might help, you need to increase prebiotics and take probiotics together, or just take prebiotics alone. I do not recommend you take probiotics alone.

Chapter 25. Dr. Bao's Weight Management Summary Recommendations

What is really special about your book?

Here is why I think my book is special. In this book, I teach:

- the scientific proved knowledge. It is obvious that if you follow the wrong beliefs, you will get wrong results.
- knowledge of food. I teach about the way of eating, and the frequency of eating.
- the skill of how to deal with hunger.
- The skill of how to deal with cravings.
- exercise. I gave you the example of what I do.
- how to prevent injury from exercise.
- how to conquer boredom.
- the skills of stress management. I found that the most important skill in the weight loss journey for most people is to master the handling of stress. Most people are handling stress by using food. In this book, I identify six main sources of stress and discuss them separately.
- the skill of keeping motivated.
- how to do environmental control (social and physical).

Why do you think your one man one book approach is better than structured multi-disciplinary lifestyle interventions?

I cannot claim that. I do have statisticians to help me with the data. I only know that I have helped hundreds of patients lose 20 lbs, 50 lbs, even 100 lbs. Their prediabetes, even diabetes, is completely reversed and fatty liver is reversed.

- Life is very complicated. Not many people can really live a structured life. We like fire fighters. Today we have to put out fire here and tomorrow there. Our daily life always changes. I want to teach people skills to handle daily challenges and become their own doctor.

- Not so many people are lucky enough to be able to get access to those so-called "structured-multidisciplinary lifestyle interventions". You have to be rich or you are lucky enough to live close to those medical centers and they are supported by US tax payer grants. Unfortunately, not so many people can move to those places. Most of my patients are struggling paying to see one doctor and certainly are not able to pay a school of specialists.
- Lifestyle change takes persistence and takes time. Most structured multidisciplinary lifestyle interventions do not last over two years because even they run out of money.
- The day comes when everyone can access a structured multi-disciplinary lifestyle intervention program. The life is the patient's life. The patient needs to make the changes. The multiple disciplinary doctor cannot live for the patient.
- I do the things I can do for my patients who might need diet education, skill improvement for stress reduction, medication adjustments, and/or physical exercise recommendations.
- Again, I think it is absurd you have to see ten different specialists, since for most people you have a life to live besides losing weight.
- Do not mistakenly think that I am against multidisciplinary or team work. My point is that every doctor should be a primary care doctor first, then with a specialty. As primary care doctors, we cannot be just a wellness doctor or serve as a dispatcher to send patients to different specialists. At least, we should be a model in terms of lifestyle and able to counsel our patients about healthy lifestyle. Again, you are lucky if your doctor can assemble a team of care for you and dose not increase the burden to an unbearable level.

What are your recommendations summarized?

I have elaborated in previous chapters. Here I summarize the key points.

- For some patients, you might just need to make one habit change.
    - I have patients who lost 20 lbs just by stopping drinking sweet tea.
    - who lost 20 lbs just by quitting drinking of a six-pack of regular soda daily.
    - who lost 20 lbs just by quitting 6-pack of beer.
    - who lost 20 lbs just by quitting a bowl of ice-cream after dinner.

  - who lost 20 lbs just by quitting eating a bag of chips after meals.
  - who lost 20 lbs just by quitting daily pancakes.
  - who lost 20 lbs just by quitting daily donuts.
  - who lost 20 lbs just by cutting their dinner portion in half.
  - who lost 10 lbs just by starting to exercise.
  - I have many other examples.
- Choose whole food/unprocessed. Choose whole grain (barley, brown rice, whole wheat, chia seeds, quinoa, bulgur, millet…), beans. Tofu is "processed" but okay.
- **Portion control is crucial**. Try to eat half what you were eating before. Especially cut your dinner by half. If you are still not losing weight, cut down your portion by another half.
- **Controlling carbs are extremely important**. We just eat too many carbs and our body do not have a chance to metabolize them. I recommend only consuming the carbs equivalent to calories you burn by exercise. For example, if you exercise and burn 400 calories, then you can have 100 g of carbs for one day (400 divided by 4=100. Every one carb has four calories). If you do not any exercise, then you need to start. Every day (except on days of sickness) we need to exercise because we eat carbs every day.
- Limit your starchy vegetables such as potatoes.
- Maximize your non-starchy vegetables intake. Expand your horizon. Try something you never tried before. Look for a good recipe in the store or online. When I first came to America, I did not know how to pronounce "asparagus," now it is my favorite. I did not know okra before, now I love it however you cook it.

Here I want to introduce a few more Chinese vegetables to you. You can buy them from an Asian store. They are delicious and affordable.

  - Bok Choy is a dark green leafy vegetable. I have a recipe in this book. You can google for more tasty recipes.
  - Winter melon is a gourd. Some people also translate it as white gourd. If you go to an Asian store, ask for winter melon and people will understand. We usually use it to make soup. It has very high dietary fiber (50%) and low carbs. It is really good to make you feel full.
  - Loofah is also a kind of gourd which was used to make sponges. It has lots of other names but we do not really know how to translate them into English. Some people also call it towel gourd, or sponge gourd. It is shaped like cucumbers.

Again, it is really good for soup. It is very tasty and makes you feel full. It has very high fiber (think about it, it was used to make sponges).

- Daikon is like carrots but white and huge. In comparison to carrot, it has much fewer carbs and so much more dietary fiber. We also use it to cook soup. It will certainly make you full with minimal calories and lots of fiber. Remember, it is very nutritious and tastes good. I have a simple recipe in this book but google for all different recipes. For some reason, I have never seen it in a Chinese restaurant.
- Hyacinth bean is very interesting. I thought it was Chinese, but I found out it was also called Indian bean or Egyptian bean. We eat it when it is young and immature. We eat the whole pod. Look for different recipes and you might like it. We stir fry with lots of garlic and at the end we just add a teaspoon of Korean soybean paste.
- Gailan is a dark green leafy vegetable. Taiwanese call it Chinese broccoli. It does not look like broccoli at all. Try it in a Chinese restaurant to see if you like it. It is very nutritional and tasty.
- Lotus root is full of nutrients. It does have some carbs but low carbs. Americans usually do not eat it. You can use it to make soup or a dish. Google a recipe.
- Cayrote is also a gourd. It has low carbs and high fiber with various nutrients. You can eat it raw in a salad or make soup or stir fry. There are many other ways to try it.

- For some people who cannot do the portion control, I recommend **intermittent fasting or meal replacement, or non-starchy vegetable only meal**, like skip or replace at least four meals a week.
- No snacking, even on fruit. Fruit has lots of fructose and can make you hungrier and gain weight.
- Do not go places where you need a lot of self-discipline to control what you eat. These places are like buffet places or bars.
- Every day fast for at least 12 hours. It is better if you can do 14 hours.
- Eating is in our genes. We like sugar (carbohydrates) which is also in our genes. This is science. Any diet which deprives a whole group of food is doomed to fail. However, employing some techniques, we can stay away from refined sugars and purified oils.
- Eating is difficult. You have to be vigilant all the time. We draw lots of pressure from eating. We celebrate everything by eating. We have birthdays, anniversaries. We eat when people are born or die. In China, people say hi by asking the question "Have you eaten your meal?" (If

you happen to visit China, when you hear this question, do not mistake it as an invitation to dinner.)

- Stress and stress responses are also in our genes. We cannot eliminate them all. However, employing some techniques, we can transform them into good outcomes.
- Any sort of activity is helpful. You can do house chores, walking, gardening. If you want to actively lose weight, it is better to do exercise while fasting, so your body has the opportunity to burn fat.
- High intensity interval training is the best way to lose weight. You can do it at any time and any place. (I only recommend you be free of cardiovascular disease.)
- For any activity, you need to start slow and build your strength slowly. Otherwise, you are going to hurt yourself and then you have an "excuse" to stop exercising.
- Exercise every day.
- Commit yourself to improve your emotional intelligence to manage your stress.

Can you tell your rationales behind your recommendations?

- Study after study has shown that long term weight loss requires a lifestyle change. It is not a crash diet. All crash diets are short-lived, since we can only live on those crash diets for a short term. I help you develop a strategy which works for you.
- All those crash diets are using the way of eliminating a whole food group. Certainly, it might help losing weight. Remember, we only have three groups of food: protein, fat and carbs. They are all vital to your life. You need them.
- Some crash diets lead people to replace one group of food with another. Before, we used carbs to replace fat. Now we use fat to replace carbs. Another outcome is the yo-yo diet. At the end, people are confused and do not know which diet to follow.
- Our body is designed to use carbohydrates first to go to energy. Fat is used as stored energy and protein is used for emergencies.
- Periods of fasting are important for weight loss. When your body has plenty of sugar, it will not use fat for energy. Fasting can lead to mild ketosis and this way is better than eliminating the whole group of carbs to force your body into ketosis, since this way increases significantly the burden on your liver and kidneys.
- Studies have revealed any attempt to replace one major macronutrient group will cause a craving rebound.

- Some crash diets eliminate all the grains and beans. Even before agriculture, humans ate wild grains. Grains and beans have multiple nutrients. I do not think it is a good idea to eliminate them all. Certainly, again portion control is crucial. Consumption needs to be matched with your physical activity.
- The key issue here is not the fat or carb itself. The key is too much in relating to our physical activity. Forty years ago, in China the main food was rice. People were eating two pounds of rice a day with no obesity, diabetes or heart disease (google "China Study"). However, at that time, people were engaged in very strenuous manual work, and we did not have heat, air conditioning, cars. Look at the Mongolians, they were eating meat all the time, but they were fit and healthy and the type 2 diabetes rate was close to zero 40 years ago. They were truly hunting and gathering. However, look at the Mongolians now. From the Mongolia Diabetes Association report in 2015 they had 7.3% prevalence rate and it was increasing.
- We are all stress eaters. Keep practicing and working on your skills to improve your emotional intelligence so you can manage your stress better and not get stuck in the stressful situations.
- Use other stress reduction methods instead of relying on eating. A better alternative is exercise like running, hiking, swimming, yoga, Tai Qi,
- It is okay to fall off the wagon but get back on as soon as you can. Do not be too frustrated with yourself. Our eating is built in our genes. It is controlled by the hypothalamus. It is unconscious. Our default is to eat as much as we can if we have the opportunity. However, we need to use our frontal lobe (area that executes reasoning and controlling) to evaluate two questions-is it nutritionally good food? Do I need it? If you do not need it even if it is nutritionally good food, you should not let the unconscious hypothalamus take over your behavior. Listen to motivational speeches often which I found to be helpful for myself. We all need to be motivated.
- Life is not easy, and we do not always know which way is best. Try to do what you can and try your best to do the job you are doing.
- Life is a marathon, not a short sprint. It is okay to make small progress day after day, and eventually you can make huge progress. If you lose one pound in a month, that is 12 pounds in a year and 60 pounds in five years.
- Our goal is not just to lose weight. We want to feel better and be healthier. The crash diet might pose harm to you. Be alert, if you do not feel good and lose weight, you need to see your doctor to make sure something else is not going on.

- Make the world around you better because of you. If you can work, go to work. If you can volunteer go volunteer.
- Eating right and exercising are not everything, and it is not easy, but they're fundamental. It takes time and work.
- Time is a choice. Time is limited for everyone. However, you can always find time to do what you want to do. Make improving your health your priority. Think about it. You need a good healthy body to enjoy the things you are working on.
- I try to treat the cause for obesity, prediabetes, diabetes, fatty liver. The causes may be different to different people. It might be stress, boredom, lack of love, lack of knowledge, this book provided all of these, and it touches every aspect of life.

When do you recommend meal replacement?

I recommend meal replacement for the following conditions:

- You are otherwise very healthy and live with someone who can help monitor your situation.
- You want to lose weight quickly for some reason other than long term health, since rapid weight loss by extreme measures usually is not sustainable, nor is it healthy.
- You understand this is a short-term fix.
- You can pay for the expensive meals.
- Sometimes I do recommend meal replacement for one meal a day for someone who wants to stay away from unhealthy food or who has been trying healthy eating and exercise but just is not losing weight.
- I also let someone who travels a lot and is not able to stay on healthy eating.
- Please read Chapter 23 again for more information.

I have been doing what you have recommended, but just do not lose weight. Is there anything else I can do?

- You might need meal replacement (intermittent fasting is a form of meal replacement), but as I said the result may be short term if the way you are doing is not sustainable. I recommend more sustainable way of meal replacement (see Chapter 23).
- You might have to consider medications, surgery or other procedures.
- You can try the following regimen:
    - Have at least 14 hours fasting daily.
    - **Exercise while fasting in the morning**.

- Reduce your breakfast and lunch further by half.
- For dinner, eat only non-starchy vegetables. If not satisfactory, I recommend shirataki miracle noodles (pasta/rice). If you still feel hungry, it is okay to add back a portion of meat.

You recommend low carb, low meat and whole food diet. What is exact difference between your diet and low carb diet?

I recommend variety of food but control portions of food which contains dense calories, so we can get plenty of micronutrients while not get excessive macronutrients like carb, fat or proteins. I see so many obese patients who have micronutrient deficiency which might cause more food craving.

I cannot control my portion. What are my options besides surgery?

As we discussed, portion control is crucial. If you can do the portion control, this is the best. You can just start to eat 50% of you are eating. However, in reality, not everybody can do it. Then you can try meal replacement (see Chapter 9).

- Skip 4-7 meals a week (skipping meals is one of the extreme meal replacement). (Be sure to discuss with your doctor).
- You can replace at least 4-7 meals a week with vegetable soup, or just vegetable salad. Be sure you are only allowed to eat no starch vegetable. No meat or fruits are consumed on those meals. If you have diabetes or other serious condition, you need physician supervision.
- I have so many people worrying about nutrition deficiency if skipping meal. If you have this strong belief, I recommend meal replacement shakes (see Chapter 9).

Chapter 26. My Patients' Survey and Testimonies

Losing weight is always very difficult and very complex. In my practice, I find some patients are able to lose weight. I have patients who were able to lose 50 lbs and up to 100 lbs. Then their diabetes medications were stopped (or just reduced to oral medication like metformin) and blood pressure medications were stopped. Some patients cannot lose weight, or they lose 5-10 lbs and then gain it back.

Over the years, while taking care of obese patients with or without diabetes, I have learned so much. In order for patients to see what other people did, I put together this survey to learn more from my patients. I only sent the survey to patients who had lost 20% of their body weight and kept it off for two years.

Tell me the top three reasons why you lost weight and what you did to keep it off this time:

1. Change of diet (100% patients). 40% patients used an App to track the calories.
2. Exercise (75% patients). 30% patients used an App to track exercise.
3. Dr. Bao changed my diabetes medications/thyroid medications.
4. Other less frequent answers like ate breakfast (10%)

Do you think that if you can lose weight, everyone else can do it?

80% answered yes. (I should have had a follow-up question for the reasons.)

Do you believe that weight loss comes by eating less and moving more?

70% of my patients said yes.

Do you believe that to lose weight you have to starve yourself?

80% thought that you needed to starve yourself to lose weight. But after losing weight now only 15% think that you need to starve yourself to lose weight.

Do you believe for weight loss to occur that you have to exercise?

85% said you need to exercise.

Do you believe weight loss requires a change in your lifestyle?

100% patients said that you have to change your lifestyle to lose weight.

Do you believe that you gained so much weight before because of your bad lifestyle and/or habits? If so, why?

80% patients attributed weight gain to bad lifestyle and habits like eating too much junk food. 20% patients blamed postmenopausal, quitting smoking, hypothyroidism, stress.

Most people have been trying to lose weight but fail by losing some weight and then gaining it back. Tell me why your previous weight loss endeavor failed:

10% this is their first endeavor.
30% attributed to medical conditions like thyroid, diabetes, polycystic ovarian syndrome (PCOS) which had not been properly managed.
60% patients attributed to the "crash diet" which is designed to work for short term.

If you tried and failed losing weight before, what did you do this time to be successful and maintain the weight loss?

60% patients replied because they were able to follow my recommendations.

30% patients attributed to a medical condition which was appropriately managed.
10% patients joined programs like Weight Watchers.

About your beliefs on weight:

Do you think your metabolism is lower than other people?

Before (Yes 90%) Now (Yes 60%)

What do you use to improve your metabolism?

60% think exercise is the best way to improve metabolism.
30% credited their changed regimen.
The rest credited weight loss itself, and better diet.

About medications:

Is there any medication that you took before that you believe lead to weight gain?

50% of the patients attributed it to diabetes medications, hormones, and anti-depression medications.
The rest of the patients did not know.

What medication are you taking, or have you taken before that you believe lead to losing weight?

60% did not know.
20% believed metformin helped them lose weight.
20% believed phentermine (Adipex-p) helped them lose weight.
Some patients believed levothyroxine helped them lose weight, and some a combination of above.
Some patients believed diabetes medications like Victoza, Trulicity helped them lose weight.

Tell us the top three benefits you have now after losing the weight:

1. 60% feel better, 30% feel better about themselves (self-image, more confident). The rest have more specifics like - able to tie their shoelaces, able to fit into their favorite dress.
2. 60% answers same as above 1; 20% breathe better, 20% no more unstable blood sugar.
3. 60% the same answers as above, the rest have more specific answers like more energy, taking less oxygen, taking less medication for blood pressure/diabetes,

Motivation:

Tell us the top three reasons/motivations for losing the weight:

1. 40% wanted to look better (self-image); 20% wanted to please their spouse (or their family members), 20% wanted to feel better; 20% wanted to be healthier (prevent diabetes);
2. 20% worried about their health; 20% wanted to get their blood sugar down; 20% didn't want to buy extra-large clothes; 20% quoted because I gave them the diagnosis of morbid obesity; the rest from number 1 or number 3.
3. 40% wanted to feel better, 40% were afraid of complications from obesity, the rest from above 1 or 2.

Tell us how you stay motivated:

Here are some answers:

- Self-esteem is so much better, and they don't want to go back.
- Want to stay feeling good.
- Keep diabetes under control and do not want to pay more for medications.
- I looked at the old extra-sized clothes, I do not want them back.
- My clothes fit so much better. I feel 100 times better.
- My husband never wanted me to be big. Now he said I look like 59 years ago when we married. I want my husband to be happy.
- I know I need to do it every day, no skipping. I just need to make it a routine.

Weight loss is not easy. During the process everyone experiences "hiccups." How do you deal with setbacks?

- I just get back on.
- I just keep going, no setbacks.
- I quickly address my "hiccups" and correct them.
- I have a supporter I can always go to.
- I know Dr. Bao wants me to weigh every day, but I do not.

About Diet:

What diet are you on to lose weight?

1. Dr. Bao's low carbs, low meat, high veggie diet, whole food-70% of patients
2. Cut out all the carbs (ketogenic diet)-20%
3. Just cut down portions
4. Weight Watchers diet
5. DASH diet
6. Mediterranean diet
7. Flexitarian diet
8. MIND diet (combination of DASH diet and Mediterranean diet)
9. South Beach diet
10. Atkins diet
11. HCG diet
12. SlimFast diet
13. Vegan diet
14. Biggest loser diet
15. Other diet
16. No specific diet (10%)

What kind of diet did you have before?

-Some tried Nutrisystem.
-Some tried "military diet" also called "egg diet."
-Some ate whatever.
-Some tried diet above 2-14.

Tell us what you ate and or drank that made you gain weight before; what habits you had before?

The list is long. I listed the most common.

- Sweets
- Fast foods
- Salty food
- Too much fruit
- Soda
- Potatoes
- Fried foods
- Beans
- Bread
- Cookies
- Pasta
- Rice
- 25% patients stated eating too much or eating all day and night

Sticking to a diet means to change your eating habits. It is not easy but what did you do to make it successful?

Here are some examples.

- Reminded myself how well I felt and how bad I felt before the weight loss.
- Everybody in my family is big. I keep motivating my children and grandchildren to follow my example.
- My husband (wife) is obese and has diabetes. I am setting the good example to him (her).
- I follow Dr. Bao's recommendation. I do it slowly. I gradually cut down my portions and stop the "bad food."
- I drink water all the time instead of eating.
- I changed my eating habits.
- Consistent and persistent.

In your opinion on your weight loss journey, what was the most difficult thing in changing your diet?

Here are some examples

- Hungry all the time

- Eating out is difficult to control
- Difficult to have portion control when eating with family and friends
- It is difficult to change the eating habit

Do you eat out a lot?

Before (how many times a week):
Most people two to three times a week. One person ate every meal in a restaurant.

Now (how many times a week): average is reduced but seems not very significantly.

About snacking, do you eat any snacks?

Yes or No   If yes continue to the next two questions.

Everyone said **yes**.

What kind of snacks do you eat? Give three examples. Tell us what you were eating and now what you replaced it with if you replaced it.

Before: chips, fried food were the most common answers. Some other answers were cake, candy, milkshakes, popcorn, peanut butter crackers, cheese, fruit.
,
Now: more patients answered all sorts of veggies (carrots, celery, cauliflower), nuts and fruit.

Do you eat night time snacks? If yes, what? Tell us what you were eating and what you are eating now.

Pretty much the same as the above question.

What is the best food you think does not contribute to weight gain?

20% of patients believe anything you eat will contribute to weight gain.
The other answers were veggies, veggie soup, tuna.

Can you share your three favorite meals with us that you believe are healthy but without weight gain? Give recipes with as much detail as possible.

20% patients answered no favorite just portion control.
The following are the common answers:

- Tuna whole wheat sandwich
- Grilled salmon with vegetables
- Turkey whole wheat sandwich
- Steamed or boiled veggies like broccoli, cauliflower, brussels sprouts, carrots
- Green salads
- Rotisserie chicken

No one gave any recipes.

Can you share with us three quick meals you go to if you do not have time to cook? Provide recipes with as much detail as possible.

All referred to above and no recipes were shared.

Do you eat fruit? If yes, how many servings do you eat every day and what do you usually eat?

20% say no.
The rest answered two to four servings of all sorts: berries, apples, bananas, watermelon, cantaloupe.

Do you eat dairy? How much every day?

60% said no.
The rest reported one cup milk in the morning, and some said ¼ cup of cheese for salad.

Do you have food cravings?

60% said yes.

How do you deal with food cravings?

20% stay busy and keep their mind off food.
20% focus on portion control.
20% focus on drink water or tea instead of eating.
20% eat healthy food like veggies, veggie soup.
20% eat nuts, fruit, or trail mix.

Food temptation is everywhere. How do you deal with temptations?

Here are some selected answers.

- Avoid places with food temptation.
- Do not bring snacks home.
- Keep telling myself if I eat, I will gain weight and increase my sugar.
- I just do not want to go back to my old me.
- Just do not start to eat.

Do you have sweet cravings?

50% sometimes

How do you deal with sweet cravings?

Here are some selected answers.

- I made a decision about how much I was going to eat before I went to the place with desserts.
- Sometimes, I eat a small portion of homemade pie.
- I eat an apple instead or other fruit.
- I drink water or tea.
- I keep myself busy and keep my mind off the sweets.

What is your weakness in dealing with eating? How did you overcome it?

Here are some examples:

Portion control: use smaller plate, eat slower, mindful eating, only fix what portion I am supposed to eat, use app to control my calories.

Food selection (eat whatever I want): follow Dr. Bao's recommendations, try not to eat if not on his list, keep practicing self-control.

Intermittent fasting: use meal replacement or vegie soup.

Are you a stress eater?

Only 50% patients say yes. (This really surprised me.)

How do you deal with stress eating?

Selected answers:

- Not to go out to eat, since usually I choose the wrong food and eat more than I needed
- Deal with stress differently, like taking a walk/go to the gym
- Drink some water instead.
- Try to eat healthier food. I try to cook for myself.

Drinks:

What do you drink now? What did you drink before?

Now: water, coffee, tea, milk
Before: sweet tea, all sorts of soda, sports drinks

How much do you drink every day?

64 oz and above.

Special Occasions:

There are a lot of free lunches--church gatherings, potlucks, parties. How do you deal with these occasions?

- 40% said they don't go to those events.

- 20% practice portion control.
- 20% only eat healthy food.
- 20% bring my own food.

I have patients who work so hard to lose weight, and then the holidays come and anniversaries or vacations. They gain all the weight back. How do you deal with these occasions?

Selected answers:

- 40% said they treated these special occasions as another regular day.
- 20% just ate less, practiced portion control.
- 20% said just get back on ASAP.
- 10% try to celebrate in different ways not just by indulging in food.

Did you change the way you celebrate?

Everybody said their way of celebrating had been changed including different healthier food, portion control and activities. One patient said that before they celebrate their anniversary by going to an expensive restaurant, now they celebrated their anniversary by having a bowling night. Another couple responded that before they hosted a party, now they just went hiking on Pinnacle Mountain.

Did you change your holiday food menu?

100% said yes. Most people said no sweets.

Did you change the way you eat during the holidays? Please specify.

- Most patients practice portion control.
- Stay away from sweets.
- Majority limit their carbohydrates.

Physical activity:

What did you do to increase your physical activity (also how much time in a week)?

40% patients go to a gym to exercise at least five days a week.
The rest just do exercise at home by walking, running, taking care of the yard, or mopping the floor. I have one patient who goes to physical therapy.

Do you think you can do more physical activities? If not, why?

80% said no. They cited time constraints and various medical conditions like COPD, severe arthritis, etc.

Do you have any advice for somebody who has not been active before?

This is actually amazing. 100% patients said you need to start **slowly** and work up **gradually** and keep the expectation **reasonable**. Most patients emphasize building a routine and not expecting results right away. It takes time.

Weight loss is a journey and everybody has a story to tell. Please share your story:

Ben:

I am Ben. I was 72 years old the first time I came to Dr. Bao for unstable blood sugar (from 40 to over 250) but with normal A1c. This had been going on for many years. No one knew what was going on with me. My own doctor was confused whether I did or did not have diabetes. My doctor also suspected that I might have pancreatic cancer. I had a CT and MRI and they found something on my pancreas but in the end, it was nothing. I felt very sluggish and depressed and frustrated. Who would not be? At my first visit, Dr. Bao reviewed my case carefully. He told me that he could solve my problem and make me feel better if I would follow what he said. He gave me a diagnosis of reactive hypoglycemia and discussed what was going in my body. Everything he explained was so clear and so logical. It made sense. He gave me his diet recommendations and also provided a handout of his diet.

I followed it religiously and miraculously my symptoms of low sugar went away, and I began to feel better. I also began to shed weight, like one pound a week. I lost 50 lbs in a year. Now it is more than two years later, and I still keep the weight off. I learned what to eat and how to eat. Dr. Bao's diet does not deprive. Just stay away from some really bad food and the rest is just portion control.

He gave me my life back.

Chris

I was 36 years old when I first saw Dr. Bao for diabetes. I had had diabetes for a few years already. It was never controlled. My A1c was over 11% and my triglycerides were over 1600. (Normal is below 150.) I was on three medications and four insulin shots. My sugar was still not able to be controlled. My weight was going up. The first visit to Dr. Bao it was 306 pounds. I felt awful. He reviewed my case and labs carefully.

He spent time discussing my diet and exercise, but most importantly my stress. He adjusted my diabetes medications. My weight came off like crazy. In a year, I lost 66 lbs. Now more than two years later, my weight is between 240 and 255. I am off all insulin shots. My sugar is stabilized and my A1c is around 5.8 %. My triglycerides were 86 in my most recent report.

Dr.Bao added years to my life and life to my years.

Callie

Now I am 80 years old, but I feel like 60 thanks to Dr. Bao. I was referred to him for controlling my diabetes five years ago. I have had diabetes for decades, and it has never been well controlled. My medication list became longer and longer. I had oral medications and injections. My weight was going up and up. At one point, I was close to 200 lbs. I am only five feet tall. I was referred to a few doctors before but without any results. Dr. Bao is different. He does not just look at your diabetes. He pays attention to other conditions that you have. In my case, he also adjusted my thyroid medication. I am following his diet and exercise recommendations which are not hard at all. My weight is coming down. I lost a wobbling 60 lbs. My family doctor began to worry and asked me to eat more food which was not on Dr. Bao's list. I told him that I feel great and I do not need more weight. Now I am off diabetes medications and I am off blood pressure medications. Thanks to Dr. Bao I gained so much more by losing so much!

Floyesia

I was referred to Dr. Bao for high calcium. I was diagnosed with primary hyperparathyroidism and eventually had surgery. My calcium was normalized. He did not stop here and discussed my weight problem. As a matter of fact, I always wanted to lose weight. I tried different diets, but nothing worked. I think partly I was so tired and not able to do so much. All the diets I was on also made me so hungry and I felt deprived.

Dr. Bao's diet is great. He just eliminates the real junk food. The rest is portion control. I always had the issue of hunger. He prescribed phentermine (½ tab) for me. I was able to stay on track. I have lost over 45 lbs and have been able to keep it off. I was wearing size 14 and now 8-10. Dr. Bao really knows what he is doing. He fixed my health first but didn't stop there. He made my life so much better.

James

I have been seeing Dr. Bao for a while. I was referred to Dr. Bao for thyroid nodules. He is also an expert on that. He examined my thyroid with ultrasound and told me that I really did not need to have a biopsy. Previously my doctor asked me to have surgery. I wanted a second opinion. This is why I was referred to Dr. Bao. I am really glad that I became Dr.Bao's patient. After he got my concerns about the thyroid nodules resolved. he began to talk to me about other aspects of life. He inquired as to what I had done to lose weight. I was really embarrassed to say that I had tried all sorts of weight loss programs on TV. I was able to lose some weight after finishing the program but gained it back and more after the program. When I saw Dr. Bao, I weighed 301 lbs, and felt tired and depressed, and mad about myself.

What I like about Dr.Bao's approach is that he was there to motivate me and cheer me every visit. The most important thing I learned from him is that weight loss is not a program you can finish. It is a lifestyle change. I suddenly realized why I had been failing all the time because I finished one program after another.

Thanks to Dr. Bao, five years later, I am 244 lbs as of today (Dec. of 2018). I lost 57 lbs. My colleagues are all very jealous and I feel fantastic. Again, I am not doing a weight program. I am just living a healthier way.

Sharon

I was referred to Dr. Bao for hypothyroidism. My weight was going up and up without stopping. It was 246 lbs. In high school, I was only 110 lbs. I do not know how I came here. I also felt terrible. I felt draggy every day. I felt embarrassed to stand by my husband who weighs only 148 lbs and is taller than I am. I also developed diabetes. I knew I could not take it anymore. Dr. Bao worked on my hypothyroidism and got it regulated. He also worked on my eating. I was a stress eater and mindless eater. He made me pay attention to what I eat. He worked on my diabetes. I was started on metformin and Victoza. My weight came down. I lost 81 lbs (now I am 165 lbs), but I want to keep going. I want to get to my husband's weight of 148 lbs. I know I can do it.

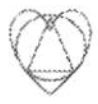

Many people asked me the meaning of the drawing on the cover.

The inner side triangle means that we need to live our lives with a purpose and wide foundation. We need to strive to do that, otherwise our lives will have lots of turmoil and stress.

The circle means everything has a reason. The circle also means that our lives are cycles. We are becoming bigger and older and eventually die. New lives are coming. Focus on next generation. Enjoy our lives with them and help young people.

The bigger heart encloses our lives. We all want to love and be loved. If we are in the heart of love, we are in peace and live the way we want to live.

You might have a better explanation. Enjoy!

56307682R00151

Made in the USA
Middletown, DE
23 July 2019